The new primary care

Modern, dependable, successful?

*Edited by Bernard Dowling
and Caroline Glendinning*

Open University Press

Open University Press
McGraw-Hill Education
McGraw-Hill House
Shoppenhangers Road
Maidenhead
Berkshire
England
SL6 2QL

email: enquiries@openup.co.uk
world wide web: www.openup.co.uk

First published 2003

A catalogue record of this book is available from the British Library

ISBN 0 335 21250 6 (pb)   0 335 21251 4 (hb)

Library of Congress Cataloging-in-Publication Data
CIP data has been applied for

Typeset by RefineCatch Limited, Bungay, Suffolk
Printed in the UK by Bell & Bain Ltd, Glasgow

Contents

List of tables and figures   viii

Acknowledgements   xi

Notes on contributors   xiii

PART 1
Primary care policies, concepts and contexts   1

1 Introduction: 'Modernizing' the NHS   3
Caroline Glendinning and Bernard Dowling

2 Primary care organizations and the 'modernization' of the
NHS   21
Matthew Bond and Julian Le Grand

3 English primary care organizations in an international context   40
Ray Robinson

4 Primary care organizations, inequalities and equity   54
Deborah Baker

5 The new institutional structures: Risks to the doctor–patient
relationship   70
Bronwyn Croxson, Brian Ferguson and Justin Keen

PART 2
Inside primary care organizations   83

6 Organizational development and governance of primary care   85
Bernard Dowling, David Wilkin and Keri Smith

7 Improving the quality of health care through clinical
governance   101
Stephen Campbell and Martin Roland

8 Information for health   123
Diane Jones and David Wilkin

9 Shifting the balance between secondary and primary care   142
Bernard Dowling and David Wilkin

10 Improving local health   159
Stephen Peckham

**11 Public involvement and democratic accountability in primary
care organizations**   179
Timothy Milewa, Stephen Harrison and George Dowswell

**12 Looking outwards: Primary care organizations and local
partnerships**   196
Caroline Glendinning, Anna Coleman and Kirstein Rummery

PART 3
Conclusions   217

13 The 'new' primary care: Ideology and performance   219
Bernard Dowling and Caroline Glendinning

Index   231

This book is dedicated to David Wilkin; without his insight into the changing picture of primary care, his vision in designing the Tracker Survey and his diligence in managing it, this book could not have been written.

Tables and figures

Tables

2.1	Ownership and governance dimensions and their ideological connotations	22
2.2	A hypothetical example of a collective decision-making problem: GPs' preferences for three clinics	30
8.1	Key targets for primary care	128
8.2	How well do information systems meet PCG/Ts' needs for information to support core functions?	134
8.3	Percentage of PCGs and PCTs reporting more than 50 per cent of practices using common information management tools in general practice	135
8.4	Access by PCG/Ts to information about general practice activity	136
8.5	Percentages of PCG/Ts expecting to meet the specified national targets (2001/2)	136
12.1	Responsibilities of social services representatives	201

Figures

2.1	Trust game	34
6.1	Organization and governance structure of primary care trusts	88
6.2	Percentages of stakeholders considered by PCG board chairs and PCT executive committee chairs to be well represented (2000/1 to 2001/2)	90
6.3	Percentages of PCG/Ts planning shifts in expenditure	96
7.1	Clinical governance in the English National Health Service	102
7.2	Percentages of PCG/Ts with strategies to implement national service frameworks in 2002	105
7.3	Percentages of PCG/Ts with individuals with lead responsibility for implementing clinical governance in areas covered by national service frameworks in 2002	106
7.4	Percentages of PCG/Ts using different strategies to implement clinical governance	106
7.5	Percentages of PCG/Ts collecting anonymous and identifiable data on general practice performance	109

7.6 Percentages of PCG/Ts using various methods for dealing with
      poor performers   110
7.7 Implementing clinical governance for coronary heart disease in a
      systems-based model   114
7.8 Reconciling quality assurance and quality improvement   116
7.9 Percentages of PCG/Ts reporting barriers to implementing clinical
      governance   116
7.10 Percentages of core general practice staff 'very supportive' or
      'supportive' of clinical governance   118
9.1 Commissioning responsibilities of PCG/Ts (2001/2)   148
9.2 Factors rated by commissioning leads as important in
      commissioning decisions (2001/2)   149
9.3 Percentages of PCG/Ts reporting integrated care pathways (2001/2) 152
9.4 Commissioning performance of PCGs and PCTs (2001/2)   154
12.1 Changes in health/social services staff   206

Acknowledgements

We would like to thank Fran Morris and Shirley Halliwell for their thoroughness and persistence in preparing the manuscript and checking references; we hope their Christmas was not spoiled. Thanks also to Ross McNally for help with bibliographic queries and to Cathy Thompson and Jacinta Evans at Open University Press for guidance and help. Above all, we would like to thank our contributors, who responded to our increasingly urgent requests with unfailing promptness, patience and good humour.

Notes on contributors

Deborah Baker has an academic background in social psychology. The focus of her research has been in epidemiology and public health, especially issues concerned with understanding and tackling health inequality. She took up the post of Professor in Public Health and Deputy Director of the Institute for Public Health Research and Policy at the University of Salford in March 2003.

Matthew Bond is a sociologist. He is Lecturer at University College London, Fellow in Primary Care at the London School of Economics and holds a research and development award from the Department of Health. His research interests include the sociology of corporate elites, the sociology of health care organizations and mathematical sociology.

Stephen Campbell is Research Fellow at the National Primary Care Research and Development Centre at the University of Manchester. His background is in public administration and health services research and his main research interests focus on the quality of care in general practice, developing and applying quality measures, and quality improvement.

Anna Coleman is Research Fellow at the National Primary Care Research and Development Centre, University of Manchester. She joined NPCRDC in January 2000, having worked in social and market research within local government for the previous 5 years. Since then she has worked on a major longitudinal survey following the development of PCG/Ts and various associated partnership projects. Her current interests include the development of health scrutiny, partnerships with local authorities, consultation with the public and the PCG/T development agenda.

Bronwyn Croxson is Senior Analyst at the New Zealand Treasury. She has been involved in economics research and teaching since 1988 and has previously held posts at the Centre for Market and Public Organization in the University of Bristol, at the School of Health Policy and Practice in the University of East Anglia, at the Institute of Child Health in University College London, and at the University of Cambridge. Her research interests centre on the application of institutional economics to public sector organizations and on the history of hospitals.

Bernard Dowling is Research Fellow in the National Primary Care Research and Development Centre at the University of Manchester. His research interests include organization and governance structures in primary care, the use of quasi-markets in public health systems, and the purchasing and commissioning of secondary care services by primary care agencies.

George Dowswell has worked in community education, the voluntary sector and management training. Following a PhD in organizational behaviour at the Management Centre, University of Bradford, he has carried out various research, evaluation and consultancy projects in the fields of health and training. He currently holds the Hallsworth Fellowship in Political Economy in the Department of Applied Social Sciences, University of Manchester.

Brian Ferguson is Professor of Health Economics and Head of Research at the Nuffield Institute for Health, University of Leeds. He has been engaged in health economics research, teaching and consultancy for approximately 17 years, 11 of which were at the University of York, latterly as Deputy Director of the Centre for Health Economics. Between 1997 and 2000 he was an Assistant Director at North Yorkshire Health Authority, with responsibility for implementing evidence-based health care. He is also a non-executive director of Selby and York Primary Care Trust and an honorary member of the Faculty of Public Health Medicine.

Caroline Glendinning is Professor of Social Policy in the National Primary Care Research and Development Centre at the University of Manchester, where she leads a programme of research on partnerships between NHS and local authority services. Her previous research has been in the fields of community care, disability and aged care, informal and family care and primary health care. She is co-editor, with Martin Powell and Kirstein Rummery, of *Partnerships, New Labour and the Governance of Welfare* (Policy Press, 2002).

Steve Harrison worked at the Nuffield Institute for Health, University of Leeds between 1978 and 2000, where he was successively Senior Lecturer in Health Policy, Reader in Health Policy and Politics, and Professor of Health Policy and Politics. He became Professor of Social Policy at the University of Manchester in 2000, where he leads the health and community research cluster in the Department of Applied Social Sciences and co-directs the innovative Masters in Research degree programme.

Diane Jones became a Fellow at the National Primary Care Research and Development Centre in 1997, where she is currently undertaking a PhD in Information Management and Technology within Primary Care Trusts. Before this Diane worked for 10 years in the National Health Service in a range of roles, including Librarian at a large teaching hospital, Information and IT Manager at a family health services authority and Primary Care IT Manager at a health authority.

Justin Keen is Professor of Health Politics and Information Management at the Nuffield Institute for Health at the University of Leeds. His main research interests are in the politics of health care and in the role of information technologies in organizational processes. He has previously worked at Brunel University, the National Audit Office and the King's Fund.

Julian Le Grand is the Richard Titmuss Professor of Social Policy at the London School of Economics. He is the author, co-author or editor of twelve books and over ninety articles and book chapters on economics and public policy, including health. He has acted as an adviser to the World Bank, the European Commission, the World Health Organization, the UK Department of Health and Social Security and the National Audit Office on health policy, welfare policy and social exclusion.

Timothy Milewa is Lecturer in sociology at the Centre for the Study of Health, Department of Human Sciences, Brunel University.

Stephen Peckham is Reader in Health Policy in the Department of Sociology and Social Policy at Oxford Brookes University. He previously worked in the voluntary and local government sectors. His research interests include health policy analysis, partnerships, public involvement, primary care and public health. Stephen is co-author, with Mark Exworthy, of *Primary Care in the UK: Policy, Organisation and Management* (Palgrave Macmillan, 2003).

Ray Robinson is Professor of Health Policy at LSE Health and Social Care, London School of Economics and Senior Fellow at the European Observatory on Health Care Systems. From 1993 to 1998 he was Professor of Health Policy and Director of the Institute for Health Policy Studies at the University of Southampton and from 1990 to 1993 he was Deputy Director of the King's Fund Institute, London. His work at LSE is concerned with various aspects of health finance, economics and management and he has published widely in this field. He has published over 150 articles and seven books on health and social policy. His most recent book (with Andrea Steiner) is *Managed Health Care: US Evidence and Lessons for the NHS* (Open University Press, 1998).

Martin Roland is Director of the National Primary Care Research and Development Centre at the University of Manchester; he is also a general practitioner in central Manchester. His particular research interest is how quality of care can be measured and improved.

Kirstein Rummery is Lecturer in health and community care in the Department of Applied Social Sciences, University of Manchester. She has previously worked as a researcher in the fields of primary health and social care, disability and citizenship, at the National Primary Care Research and Development Centre and the Universities of Birmingham and Kent, and has published widely in these areas.

Keri Smith is a Research Associate at the National Primary Care Research and Development Centre. A core member of the National Tracker Survey management team, she has particular interests in governance, stakeholder involvement and organizational development. Currently, Keri's research interests include the impact of culture on general practice and ethnographic methodologies.

David Wilkin is Emeritus Professor of Health Services Research at the University of Manchester. He designed and directed the National Tracker Survey of Primary Care Groups and Trusts and was the founding director of the National Primary Care Research and Development Centre. His research in primary health care has focused on policy implementation and the organization and delivery of services.

PART 1
Primary care policies, concepts and contexts

1 Introduction: 'Modernizing' the NHS

Caroline Glendinning and Bernard Dowling

Introduction: New Labour and the 'modernization' of the NHS

Since coming to power in 1997, the Labour government has placed the National Health Service (NHS) at the heart of a concerted drive to 'modernize' public sector services. 'Modernization' is a loose term that is capable of multiple meanings and interpretations and that also has significant normative overtones – who would eschew modernization in favour of 'old-fashioned' or 'outdated' public services? Modernization is perhaps most commonly used to refer to the process of updating services to match the expectations of contemporary publics or consumers. This may include attempts to tackle complex and long-standing social problems, such as the causes of avoidable morbidity and mortality and the wide variations in the use and experiences of health services by different sectors of the population. Modernization is also an implicit response to the challenges posed by economic globalization, in that it acknowledges the importance of maximizing efficiency in the use of public resources to sustain economic competitiveness. It therefore has the potential to open up to change those parts of the public sector that remained untouched, or failed to be transformed, by the market ethos of previous Conservative governments. This can involve challenging some cherished traditions and vested interests, such as those of professional groups who may attempt to protect their remaining autonomous domains from rationalizing managerial influences (Newman 2000, 2001).

However, unlike the politics of its immediate predecessors, who regarded taxation and public expenditure as more or less negative influences on economic competitiveness and who therefore sought to prioritize efficiency and value for money over most other concerns, the Labour government's 'modernization' agenda also embraces a concern for social, moral and civic values. It therefore includes a strong appeal to principles of consensus and social inclusion, and an awareness of the roles – both actual and symbolic – that high-quality public welfare services can play in building and sustaining social cohesion. Thus the continuing drive to improve efficiency is now accompanied by equally urgent pressures to improve the quality and responsiveness of services to improve outcomes for the individuals who use them.

Underpinning Labour's 'modernization' project is the articulation of a 'Third Way', a pragmatic political paradigm that involves taking the 'best' (however defined) of both traditional, hierarchical, state-based welfare and more recent market approaches to social policy and building on these (Giddens 1998). Indeed, it has been argued that the Labour government's appropriation of the term 'modernization' itself draws on several different traditions and meanings that incorporate both earlier and more recent conceptions of the contemporary state (Newman 2001). Thus, for example, since the government's first 2 years in office during which it adhered to the public expenditure plans of the previous Conservative administration, very substantial amounts of new funding have been injected into key areas of public sector services. For 20 years before 1997, annual real terms growth in spending on the NHS had remained at around 3 per cent ('real terms' growth is the extra money available, relative to the expansion of the economy, with pay and prices held broadly constant). However, between 1997 and 2001, annual real terms growth in NHS spending doubled to 6.1 per cent (Jones 2001). Further increases in funding for the NHS were announced in the 2001 and the 2002 budgets, taking annual real terms growth to 7.4 per cent for the years 2002/3 to 2007/8. This level of real terms growth in NHS funding is almost three times higher and has been committed for a longer period than for the public sector as a whole; other public sector real terms growth remains at 2.5 per cent for only the 2 years 2004/5 and 2005/6 (HM Treasury 2002). In cash terms, the additional investment announced in the 2002 budget increased total spending on the NHS across the UK from £65.4 billion in 2002/3 to a projected £105.6 billion in 2007/8. Indeed, Paton (2002) has claimed that the most significant point in the evolution of Labour's health policy occurred with the announcement of these new spending plans: 'the message was clear: the jewel in New Labour's crown, the NHS, required significant polishing' (p. 127).

Although this level of investment bears a remarkable resemblance to 'old' Labour expenditure patterns, which privileged state over other forms of welfare, the conditions attached to these new resources and the ways in which they are to be spent reflect definitively 'new' Labour ways of governing. These ways include highly prescriptive approaches to the performance, delivery and results of public sector services. Indeed, the government has tied its electoral fortunes tightly to the attainment of these results: 'New Labour has probably set itself more targets than any previous government in history ... It has manufactured huge amounts of ammunition either to fire a celebratory salute or to shoot itself in the foot' (Powell 2002: 7).

Chapter 2 expands on these points, describing in more detail Labour's 'Third Way' philosophy and suggesting some potential implications of this philosophy for the government's attempts to reform the NHS. In this chapter, the government's ambitions for the NHS, the development of these policies and their implementation since 1997 are first described. We then explain the foundations on which these plans have been built – the legacies of the previous government's quasi-market reforms and, in particular, the growing involvement of front line health professionals, such as general practitioners, in the processes of shaping services, ensuring cost-effectiveness, safeguarding quality and managing budgets. We go on to discuss the challenges of evaluation and the concept of success in the context of these reforms. This discussion is significant, given the Labour government's proclaimed pragmatic commitment to building on 'what works'. Should the performance and outcomes of a 'modernized' NHS be measured against the objectives that the government has itself set, for example, or against some external criteria – and, if so, what? Finally, we describe the rationale and organization of the rest of the book.

Labour's reforms: the 'modernization' of the NHS

Just 7 months after coming to power in 1997, the Labour government published a White Paper setting out its plans for the reform of the NHS (Secretary of State for Health 1997). *The New NHS: Modern, Dependable* began with a clear exposition of 'Third Way' philosophy:

> In paving the way for the new NHS the Government is committed to building on what has worked but discarding what has failed. There will be no return to the old centralized command and control systems of the 1970s . . . But nor will there be a return to the divisive internal market system of the 1990s . . . Instead there will be a 'Third Way' of running the NHS – a system based on partnership and driven by performance.
>
> (Secretary of State for Health 1997: 10)

The main structural changes proposed in the 1997 White Paper were: the abolition of general practitioner (GP) fundholding, in which some individual general practices or groups of practices held budgets to purchase a limited range of hospital and other health services for their patients; and the abolition of the internal market that had been introduced into the NHS in 1991. In relation to this latter proposal, the formal separation between the purchasers and the providers of services was retained, but competition was to be replaced by collaboration; indeed, all NHS bodies were to be placed under a new statutory duty to work in partnership with each other and with other organizations. These transformed relationships would be underpinned by agreements, rather than annual contracts, governing the provision of services. Responsibility for 'commissioning' (broadly, planning and procuring services within an agreed budgetary framework) would increasingly lie in the hands of entirely new organizations – primary care groups (PCGs) and primary care trusts (PCTs). Primary care groups and trusts (PCG/Ts) would bring together GPs, community health services and other local health providers within a single organizational framework, and would be responsible for an integrated budget amounting to three-quarters of all NHS expenditure.

Primary care groups and trusts were – and remain – the organizational centrepiece of the new government's NHS reforms. They represent a major innovation and undertaking within the NHS. Each PCG/T includes all the GPs within a locality, unlike fundholding which had been optional. Typically, a PCG/T would, according to the White Paper, include around 50 GPs and approximately 100,000 registered patients (no evidence was cited to justify this size). Primary care groups and trusts have three main areas of responsibility:

- To improve the health of local people and reduce inequalities, in relation to both the risks of poor health and the use of health services. Primary care groups and trusts are responsible, in close collaboration with local author- ities and other local partner organizations, for drawing up a health improvement plan for the locality. This plan sets targets for reducing avoidable morbidity and the measures by which these targets are to be attained.
- To develop primary and community health services for the locality. This includes creating comprehensive, integrated local services out of the GP- based services that have hitherto remained largely separate, both from each other and from the community health services that, since the early 1990s, have been part of provider trusts.
- To commission hospital and community health services. This responsi- bility builds on the experiences of GP fundholding and other variants of GP-led commissioning that had developed during the internal market.

The 1997 White Paper anticipated that there would be four levels of PCG/ Ts, characterized by increasing levels of devolved autonomy and independ- ence. At level 1, PCGs would simply advise health authorities on commission- ing services. Level 2 PCGs would have devolved responsibility for the budget for purchasing hospital and community health services for their patients, again operating as subcommittees of their health authorities. At the third level, PCGs would become trusts – free-standing NHS bodies, responsible both for their own budgets and for commissioning services. At level 4, PCTs would also manage and provide a range of community health services, such as district nursing, health visiting and specialist nursing services. At levels 3 and 4, PCTs would have full responsibility for managing their budgets and would be accountable for their actions through mainstream NHS performance management arrangements.

The governance arrangements of PCG/Ts reflected this evolving status. The twelve-member boards of PCGs were dominated by primary care professionals – up to seven GPs and two nurses, with the GP members having the right to select the board chair. Other board members included a representative from the local social services department, a health authority representative and a lay representative from the local community. The PCG board formed the basis of the professional executive committee of the PCT – but, significantly, without an overall GP majority. Like other NHS trusts, PCTs also have boards, most of whose members are lay, non-executive members. However, unlike other NHS trusts, it is the PCT professional executive committee that is responsible for the formulation and implementation of local strategies and priorities; the PCT board has only oversight, not policy-making responsibilities (see Chapter 6 for further details).

A highly significant innovation was to give PCG/Ts a (notional or actual, depending on the level of PCG/T) budget that consists of a 'single cash limited envelope' (Secretary of State for Health 1997: 37). This is made up of three previously separate funding streams that had covered, respectively, spending on hospital and community health services; GP drug prescribing; and the cash-limited budget that had funded the infrastructure costs of GP practices – facilities such as premises, ancillary nursing and clerical staff, and computer systems. (The non-cash-limited budget covering remuneration for individual GPs was not included.) Integrating these formerly separate budgets offered the opportunity to make strategic shifts in resources and investment between areas of primary care provision that had hitherto been separately funded from entirely different budgets. Equally significantly, this 'single envelope' budget was determined in advance, rather than being demand-led and therefore largely open-ended. At the same time, it was announced that the basis for calculating the overall budget for primary health services across a locality or region would be altered. The traditional mode of reimbursing individual, independent contractor GPs meant that spending on primary care was heavily influenced by factors such as the number of GPs in a locality, the demands of patients, and the variable behaviours of individual GPs in prescribing, ordering diagnostic tests and referring patients to specialist hospital services. The resources allocated for general practice were, therefore, substantially demand-led and, over time, this had led to an inequitable geographical distribution of resources. Instead, the intention was to move towards a situation in which the resources allocated to PCG/Ts reflect the health needs of their populations, through the application of a new 'weighted capitation' formula that takes into account the demographic and socio-economic characteristics of the population covered by the PCG/T.

The White Paper also emphasized the importance of accountability in the 'new' NHS – not in the wider sense of public, democratic accountability, but a much narrower, managerial accountability (Rouse and Smith 2002). Two new national bodies were established. The National Institute for Clinical Excellence would set national standards and benchmarks to reduce the widespread variations in professional practices and treatments that traditionally characterized the behaviours of autonomous, independent GPs and that had arguably increased during the 1990s. The Commission for Health Improvement (subsequently to become the Commission for Health Care Audit and Inspection) would ensure that these standards and benchmarks were adhered to, through a rolling programme of inspections. The White Paper also promised the publication of national service frameworks, to establish benchmarks for the treatment of particular common conditions or patient groups. Meanwhile, measures to safeguard the quality of primary care services were built into the responsibilities of PCG/Ts through the concept of 'clinical governance'. This was intended to 'build on and strengthen the existing systems of professional self-regulation and the principles of corporate governance', by requiring 'practitioners to accept responsibility for developing and maintaining standards within their local NHS organizations' (Secretary of State for Health 1997: 47). These measures threatened to encroach on cherished clinical freedoms, through the introduction of increasing specification, standardization and centralization (Harrison 2002). Their presentation was, however, accompanied by eloquent appeals to the importance of equity and fairness; an end to the variations in patients' experiences that had characterized the former internal market; and the re-creation of a one-nation NHS. At the same time, an array of new performance targets were introduced, including waiting times for access to primary and secondary health services, improvements in patient satisfaction, reductions in avoidable morbidity and good performance benchmarks.

The White Paper's emphasis on managerial accountability was nevertheless complemented and, indeed, justified by the need to improve relationships between the NHS and the general public to rebuild public confidence; 'the NHS, as a public service for local communities, should be both responsive and accountable' (Secretary of State for Health 1997: 29). Public involvement in the development of health improvement programmes and in the activities of PCG/Ts was therefore promised, as were new surveys of patient and user experiences.

The proposals in *The New NHS: Modern, Dependable* (Secretary of State for Health 1997) applied only to England. Different variants were proposed in subsequent White Papers covering Wales, Scotland and Northern Ireland. In Wales, the members of local health groups were to offer GPs and other frontline professionals the opportunity to influence service commissioning, again using indicative cash-limited budgets (Secretary of State for Wales 1998). Scottish plans proposed the establishment of local health cooperatives, with membership by GPs remaining optional. Vertical separations – between purchasing and provision and between primary and secondary services – were to be maintained through the creation of primary care trusts (responsible for primary health care, community hospitals and mental health services) and area health boards responsible for commissioning acute services (Secretary of State for Scotland 1998). A consultation document, *Fit for the Future* (Secretary of State for Northern Ireland 1998), set out two options for Northern Ireland. One of these resembled the proposals for PCG/Ts in England (with the additional inclusion of social services staff among the primary care professionals to whom responsibilities were to be devolved); the other option involved separating purchasers and providers through the respective operational elements of primary care partnerships and provider bodies.

Despite the differences in the proposed organizational configurations, and the time-scales for implementing these, in all four countries much emphasis was placed on the role of primary care (Rummery 1998; Exworthy 2001). This commonality led one commentator to conclude that it was unlikely 'that Scotland and Wales will develop significantly different models of care from those used in England' (Owen 1998: 9). Nevertheless, distinct variations can be seen in the organizational templates proposed for the different countries of the UK that reflect their individual political climates (Greer 2001). Moreover, the powers of territorial Parliaments and Assemblies (particularly in Scotland) to make further changes raise questions about the scope of a 'one-nation' NHS. In the longer term, devolution may well generate greater spatial variations and reduce similarities across the four countries of the UK. The focus of this book, however, is on the implementation of the NHS reforms in England, to which we now return.

In April 1999, not quite 2 years after Labour came to power, 481 PCGs covering the whole of England went 'live'. Initially, all PCGs operated at levels 1 or 2. In April 2000, the first 17 PCTs were created, with a further 23 in October 2000 and 164 in April 2001. However, in July 2000, the government unexpectedly re-launched its policy for the NHS with the publication of *The NHS Plan: A Plan for Investment, A Plan for Reform* (Secretary of State for Health 2000). This document, applicable only to England, indicated both the extent of the government's impatience with the pace of change and its growing enthusiasm for attaching performance 'strings' to new investment. *The NHS Plan* signalled further 'modernizing' changes, such as the breaking down of traditional professional role demarcations and the creation of new points of access to NHS services. However, it did not fundamentally alter the structure, roles and responsibilities of PCG/Ts. Instead, it contained numerous proposals for performance monitoring, audit and management that would be applied to

PCG/Ts and their constituent elements. *The NHS Plan* effectively endorsed and elaborated an extensive system of benchmarking and performance management, with sanctions at the end of the line if necessary, in a renewed drive to raise standards and ensure these were met (Paton 2002).

Both *The NHS Plan* and the publication in 2001 of *Shifting the Balance of Power in the NHS* (Department of Health 2001) reasserted and strengthened the role of PCG/Ts within the NHS. In the latter policy document, the 1997 intentions of devolving responsibility to locality-based PCGs and PCTs were finally realized. Health authorities, which had continued to support PCGs and manage the performance of PCTs, were to be abolished in April 2002. They would be replaced by a smaller number of strategic health authorities, covering larger areas and responsible for managing the performance of all local NHS organizations, including PCTs. At the same time, all remaining PCGs would become freestanding trusts, regardless of their current level of organizational development. This accelerated organizational transformation allowed the government to claim that by April 2002, 75 per cent of the entire NHS budget for England was devolved to local, primary care-based organizations, governed by doctors and nurses, with responsibilities for securing the provision of a full range of health services for their registered patient populations and for the management, development and integration of all primary care services (Secretary of State for Health 2002).

This organizational restructuring was, therefore, both radical and rapid. Within the history of the NHS as a whole and primary care in particular, the establishment of PCG/Ts has the potential to effect the most far-reaching transformation since its creation in 1948. Primary care groups and trusts constitute a framework within which the primary health services provided by the independent, small businesses of general practice can become part of a single, integrated system of primary care, alongside the larger, more hierarchical organizations of community health services. This does not simply mean that general practice and other non-hospital health services have become part of a single organizational and managerial framework (though this is undoubtedly an important part of the story). Rather (and as the next section of this chapter will show), PCG/Ts were also intended to build on both some of the traditional professional autonomy of general practice and on the experiences of the more entrepreneurial fundholding GPs during the years of the internal market (Ennew *et al.* 1998). This immediately suggests the potential for tensions to arise between traditional professional clinical freedoms; the extended and enhanced autonomy that had been offered to GPs under the former fundholding regime; and a new organizational framework that provides unprecedented opportunities for more tightly managed modes of planning, organizing and delivering health services, controlling costs and ensuring quality. It also suggests the possibility of tensions arising between local, parochial priorities and concerns and attempts to re-create a strong, well-performing 'national' health service, with all the overtones of equity and inclusiveness that this implies. Additionally, it indicates a potential clash between the rhetoric of devolution and strengthened frontline professional influence and the achievement of national standards through measures such as national service frameworks and tight performance assessment frameworks for PCTs. In other words, any autonomy experienced by PCTs has to be earned (Lee and Woodward 2002). How these various tensions develop and are resolved is crucial to the success of PCG/Ts; they therefore constitute major themes of this book.

Interest in the success of the PCG/T experiment is not just local. Pressures to contain public expenditure, while responding to the twin challenges of globalization and demographic change, are common to other post-industrial societies and prompt searches for new ways to improve the efficiency, quality and accountability of their welfare services. Initiatives by governments that attempt to do this, at the same time as containing the potential escalation of health care costs, are particularly important in this context. As will be shown in Chapter 3, the experiences of PCG/Ts are of wider interest, extending well beyond the shores of the British Isles.

Despite the rhetoric of incoming governments wishing to stamp a new distinctive mark on the institutions and processes they have inherited, substantial elements of continuity with previous administrations and policies are usually apparent. The NHS is no exception to this. Indeed, the rhetoric of *The New NHS: Modern, Dependable* made a positive virtue out of such continuity, through its stated intention of building on 'what works'. Thus, despite the White Paper's outright rejection of the divisive consequences of the internal market and GP fundholding, this immediate past history nevertheless provided an essential foundation on which Labour's reforms could be constructed. In the next section of this chapter, this history is briefly described. The account will highlight both the negative elements that the incoming Labour government sought to abandon or modify and the positive elements on which it hoped to build.

Background: the problem of general practice and the legacy of the internal market

Two particular policy themes are highlighted here: the experience of the internal market and the role of GP fundholders within this; and the introduction of managerial constraints on the clinical and economic behaviours of independent contractor GPs and the small business-style practices they operated.

The introduction of the 'internal market' into the NHS by Margaret Thatcher's government in April 1991 aimed radically to change a health service in which hitherto hierarchical, 'command and control' systems of accountability had been combined with very considerable professional autonomy (and, therefore, also considerable command over resources) on the part of clinicians. Although GPs did not hold quite such high status as hospital doctors, they nevertheless continued to enjoy a strongly cherished tradition of autonomy and independence (Pater 1981). The internal market sought to reduce the relative power of hospitals and enhance the power of GPs through three main mechanisms. First, the internal market separated the functions of purchasing and providing services; secondly, it introduced competition between providers to improve efficiency; and, thirdly, it built on the traditional 'gatekeeping' role of GPs and gave them a greater role in the procurement of local health services (Robinson and Le Grand 1994; Dowling 2000).

The internal market assigned to local health authorities responsibility for purchasing services from hospital and community provider organizations (NHS Trusts). However, an initially small number of individual general practices (GP 'fundholders') were allowed to hold delegated budgets with which they could purchase a limited range of hospital services for their patients. During the first half of the 1990s, the range of services that fundholders could purchase was widened and the number of GPs joining the scheme also increased, as initial restrictions on entry were relaxed and new incentives to join were introduced. By the time GP fundholding was abolished in March 1999, around 60 per cent of the population of England were patients of fundholding GPs. Despite the extended coverage of fundholding, however, health authorities maintained responsibility for purchasing most hospital and community health services.

Alongside these two main purchasing arrangements, other hybrid forms developed. A few total purchasing pilot projects, involving large general practices or groups of practices, were given extended budgets to purchase a much wider range of health services than those covered by the standard fundholding scheme. Although one of the main intentions of total purchasing pilots was to extend the opportunities for GPs to exercise purchasing leverage over acute hospital and other health services (NHS Executive 1994), their most marked achievements were in moving resources and services from hospitals to community and primary care, and in developing services based in and around general practice (Mays *et al.* 1998). Other innovations included multi-funds, in which groups of fundholding practices (rather than individual practices) joined together to purchase hospital and community health services on behalf of all their patients. Meanwhile, in some areas GPs opposed to the principles underpinning fundholding worked together as locality commissioning groups to advise their local health authorities on purchasing decisions, but without any devolution of budgetary control to the group (Regen *et al.* 1998).

It was from these arrangements that the Labour government's reforms evolved. In opposition, the Labour Party had remained implacably opposed to GP fundholding (Labour Party 1993), on the grounds that this created inequities within the NHS and generated expensive bureaucracy and red tape ('transaction costs') that diverted resources from direct patient care. Indeed, although much of the early evidence for this assertion was anecdotal, later research did show that fundholding patients tended to have significantly shorter waiting times for access to elective surgery at hospitals (Dowling 1997, 1998). The risk of increased inequities also threatened relationships between primary health and other service providers. For example, some of the total purchasing pilots used their enhanced budgetary flexibilities to improve patients' access to social services by contributing to the employment of practice-based care managers. However, local authority social services departments were anxious about participating in projects that enhanced access to services for only some of their local populations (Bosanquet 1998).

Labour was faced with a dilemma. Many GPs had become committed to the fundholding scheme (Ham 1996) and abolishing fundholding without giving GPs a central role in any new arrangement could have put the government at odds with an important section of the medical profession, a scenario most administrations would wish to avoid (Dowling 2000). Moreover, the commissioning role of GPs had indeed increased their leverage over hospital services (Klein 1995). There was a growing body of evidence that the purchaser–provider split, including fundholding, had brought some important benefits to the wider NHS, in particular the development of new services in primary care, improved efficiency and savings, and some improvements in access to specialist hospital services (Le Grand *et al.* 1998; Dowling 2000). From the various GP-dominated purchasing and commissioning arrangements that had developed under the Thatcher and Major governments, Labour therefore saw the potential for commissioning organizations in which GPs had a lead role. It is unlikely that the establishment of PCG/Ts would ever have been considered had it not been for the experience of the internal market and GP fundholding (Dowling 2000).

This experience provided the empirical justification for the incoming government's rhetoric of building on what works. Moreover, given continuing pressures to contain costs, there was no rationale for returning to a situation where GPs could make clinical decisions without also taking responsibility for their financial consequences. This can be seen as part of a longer-term trend across the public sector as a whole, in which market mechanisms are increasingly used to harness professional decision-making to financial controls (Clarke and Newman 1997). A major circle that the new Labour government attempted to square through the creation of PCG/Ts was the abolition of GP fundholding, while at the same time ensuring that GPs retained a major role in systems of resource allocation and cost control.

The creation of PCG/Ts was not the only mechanism available to the incoming government to bring about change in the English NHS, although it was certainly the most extensive and radical. Two other levers, both of which had been used by previous administrations, also had the potential to transform traditional modes of providing primary and community health services. One was the introduction of an alternative to the traditional GP contract. Even the previous Conservative government had become increasingly concerned about the wide variations in the range and quality of primary health services that had been further exacerbated by GP fundholding. The individualistic culture and existing contractual framework of general practice provided little opportunity for NHS managers to intervene to improve equity, quality or service integration. Moreover, consultation with grassroots health professionals revealed demands by GPs for greater flexibility and diversity of employment arrangements; to these arguments were added concerns about an impending crisis in the primary care workforce supply. The 1997 NHS (Primary Care) Act, passed just before the May general election, therefore introduced for the first time an alternative to the traditional GP contract – the personal medical services contract. This offers the opportunity for the much tighter contractual specification of primary care services. This might involve the targeting of services at particular areas or population groups (for example, homeless people or ethnic minority groups) for whom provision is currently poor. Personal medical services contracts can include specified standards of services. They also offer opportunities to introduce greater flexibility between the roles and responsibilities of GPs, nurses and other health professionals. Personal medical services schemes have proved popular with NHS managers and GPs alike – for the latter, they offer opportunities for more flexible salaried employment arrangements. Since April 2002, personal medical services contracts have been held by PCTs, thereby allowing PCTs to direct primary care services to disadvantaged neighbourhoods or patient groups within their locality. Furthermore, the 1997 Act laid the ground for the integration of the previously separate funding streams for GP and other community and hospital services, which was later completed through the creation of PCG/Ts.

The other mechanism that has the potential to bring about widespread changes, especially in the balance between managerial and professional interests, is the changing nature of the contract under which GPs provide general medical services to the NHS. A new contract was imposed on GPs in 1990, which, for the first time, specified minimum standards of service and tied some elements of GPs' remuneration more closely to the provision of certain services. During 2001, discussions began between the profession's leaders and the Department of Health about a revised contract – with GP practices rather than individual practitioners – that would include major new incentives to improve the quality of primary health care, as reflected in clinical processes, patients' experiences and the internal organization of practices. Under the proposed new contract, a very substantial proportion of GPs' income could be linked to the attainment of quality targets (depending on the number and complexity of these targets and the level of financial incentives on offer). The new contract is also likely to include the flexibility for individual practices to opt in or out of providing particular services, subject to negotiation with their PCT (NHS Confederation 2002). A new GP contract, therefore, has the potential to strengthen dramatically the managerial levers available to PCTs, especially in relation to their responsibilities for clinical governance (see Chapter 7).

The challenges of judging 'success' in the modernized NHS

The ambitiousness and complexity of the Labour government's objectives for primary health services make evaluation difficult. However, the government itself has highlighted the importance of evaluation and related research activities, through its promotion of evidence-based policy and practice. Indeed, the 1997 White Paper opened with the pragmatic dictum that 'what counts is what works' (Secretary of State for Health 1997: 10). Commentators have pointed out that the promotion of evidence-based policy-making is far from new (Harrison 1998; Nutley and Webb 2000). However, both what counts as evidence and the creation and implementation of policies based on 'evidence' are invariably equivocal and contested. Certain kinds of evidence tend to be privileged over others, especially quantifiable evidence that is readily and quickly available and is employed within a positivist paradigm. Klein (2000) has drawn attention to the 'attempt by the EBM [evidence-based medicine] movement to privilege certain types of evidence, notably the results of randomized trials, over other kinds of knowledge or understanding. The former is "science"; the others are not' (p. 65). This trend is, arguably, reinforced by the growing need for evidence that can underpin managerial strategies for regulating and improving performance (Ferlie *et al.* 1996). In contrast, 'evaluation of organizational restructuring or models of service delivery is methodologically more uncertain, less rigorously executed or frequently omitted' (Davies and Nutley 2000: 59). Moreover, Klein (2000) argues that the attempt to derive and apply the same evidence-based paradigm to policy-making rests on a 'gross misunderstanding of the policy process, as well as on an exaggerated claim about what research can deliver' (p. 65).

Policy innovations are themselves modified in the course of implementation, which can often extend over a considerable period. Organizational reconfigurations take time to achieve; changes in the roles, behaviours and attitudes of frontline healthcare staff and other professionals may also be required and these are likely to take even longer. Detecting change over a relatively short time-scale, when some of these changes are still incomplete, can therefore be difficult. For example, policies and practices that aim to improve population health or reduce health inequalities are likely to involve long-term programmes, the impact of which may not be detectable for up to a generation; more immediate process measures may need to be used instead (Exworthy and Berney 2000).

Furthermore (and leaving aside the impact of other levers for change, such as personal medical services contracts), the establishment of PCG/Ts, the objectives they are required to achieve and the variety of methods that are likely to be employed in addressing those objectives together make up a multi-faceted and highly complex programme of change. Success in one area (for example, reducing inequalities in access to primary care services) may be accompanied by failure to meet targets in another (for instance, reducing waiting times for hospital appointments and treatments). It may not be feasible, either practically or theoretically, to weigh up these different outcomes against each other. Evaluating complex programmes of change also generates difficulty in attributing causality. 'When a particular effect or impact is identified, how can the evaluator decide which reform facet or component produced it?' (Pollitt 1995: 139).

A further question is that of the criteria against which 'success' should appropriately be measured. Powell (2002) makes the important distinction between intrinsic and extrinsic evaluation: 'The former is based on assessing progress in terms of the government's own stated objectives . . . The latter examines a standard set of evaluation criteria, irrespective of a government's stated objectives' (p. 4). Intrinsic evaluation is therefore based on comparing stated aims and objectives with achievements, while extrinsic evaluation involves some external reference point (which may be different from the government's own objectives and, indeed, may not be accepted as legitimate by government).

As the contributions to this book will describe, in the short time since PCG/Ts were created, they have been set an extremely challenging programme of extensive and rapid organizational and cultural change. Each of the three original core functions of PCG/Ts (improving health, developing primary and community health services, and commissioning specialist health and other services) could itself be broken down into numerous smaller, or interim, goals and targets. These might also embrace less tangible objectives, such as involving frontline health professionals in all areas of strategic decision-making, engaging with local publics and communities, or working in partnership with other organizations. Actions that are directed towards one particular objective may also, indirectly or directly, contribute towards the achievement of others. For example, the appropriate commissioning of health services by PCG/Ts may also contribute towards reducing health inequalities (or, at least, reducing inequalities in experiences of health care). Conversely, some goals, and the management of performance towards achieving them, may be incompatible, or at least risk creating tensions and 'perverse incentives'. For example, enhancing the role of frontline professionals in decision-making is likely to highlight particular local needs and priorities and these may conflict with the re-creation of a one-nation NHS. Eventual outcomes are therefore likely to be long-term, multiple and potentially contradictory.

The contributors to the remainder of Part 1 of this book focus on some of the wider implications and challenges prompted by the 'new' NHS. Together, they set the Labour government's reforms within a broader context and offer a range of extrinsic criteria and analytic frameworks within which the empirical evidence presented in Part 2 can be located and interpreted. In Chapter 2, Bond and Le Grand discuss the potential for using a mix of hierarchical and market mechanisms which are associated with the 'Third Way' to achieve change in health care and services. In Chapter 5, Croxson, Ferguson and Keen address the theme of transforming relationships between professionals (particularly GPs), and between professionals and users of health services. Implicit in both chapters are the potential tensions between professional authority and autonomy (and the consequent structuring of relationships with patients) and the new forms of managerial accountability that professionals are also expected to incorporate into their own behaviours. In Chapter 4, Baker describes some of the challenges likely to be experienced by PCG/Ts in improving the health of local populations and in demonstrating such improvements. In Chapter 3, Robinson locates the English PCG/T experiment within an international context; as perhaps the most ambitious and complex organizational integration of primary care in developed economies, its outcomes will be awaited with interest.

The chapters in Part 2 of the book present detailed evidence on the operation of PCG/Ts in relation to their main objectives. The focus in each chapter is on the barriers and opportunities that are likely to affect the success, or otherwise, of these new organizations. Thus in Chapter 6, Dowling, Wilkin and Smith evaluate the development of PCG/Ts' organizational capacity and their management of the new, integrated budgets. In Chapter 7, Campbell and Roland assess the strategies used by PCG/Ts to implement clinical governance and reflect on the likely effectiveness of these strategies. Most of the responsibilities with which PCG/Ts are charged depend on the effective use of information management and technology (IM&T), a subject that Jones and Wilkin examine in Chapter 8. Chapter 9, by Dowling and Wilkin, explores how far PCG/Ts have been able to build on the experience and successes of GP fundholding in commissioning hospital services. Chapters 10, 11 and 12 take a slightly broader perspective of PCG/T activities, focusing respectively on activities to improve health and reduce health inequalities; the involvement of local communities and the general public in the decision-making of PCG/Ts; and PCG/Ts' 'partnerships' with other statutory, voluntary and private organizations.

Most of the chapters in Part 2 draw on data from the National Tracker Survey of PCG/Ts, a longitudinal survey of PCG/Ts carried out between 1999 and 2002 at the National Primary Care Research and Development Centre at the University of Manchester (Wilkin *et al.* 1999, 2001, 2002). The Tracker Survey was originally based on a representative sample of 15 per cent (72) of PCG/Ts (some subsequently merged). Three separate 'sweeps' of the survey were carried out, approximately 6 months, 18 months and 3 years after PCG/Ts came into being. The fieldwork for the first 'sweep' involved interviews with PCG chief officers, chairs and health authority leads; and postal questionnaires to clinical governance, prescribing, IM&T leads, social services representatives on PCG boards, and other GP and nursing board members. Fieldwork for the two subsequent 'sweeps' of the Tracker Survey followed the same pattern, although the face-to-face interviews were replaced by telephone interviews.

Large and complex surveys of this kind have their limitations, especially in the level and depth of detail they are able to collect. However, the Tracker Survey provides a unique picture of a process of major organizational development from the different perspectives of several key stakeholders. Being able to offer a multi-faceted, pluralistic account is a major strength in research on complex organizational change and this will, we hope, also be reflected in the remainder of this book.

References

Bosanquet, N. (1998) *The Bromsgrove Total Purchasing Project 1994–8*. London: Imperial College School of Medicine.

Clarke, J. and Newman, J. (1997) *The Managerial State*. London: Sage.

Davies, H. and Nutley, S. (2000) Healthcare: evidence to the fore, in H.T.O. Davies, S.M. Nutley and P.C. Smith (eds) *What Works? Evidence-based Policy and Practice in Public Services*. Bristol: Policy Press.

Department of Health (2001) *Shifting the Balance of Power in the NHS*. London: Department of Health.

Dowling, B. (1997) Effect of fundholding on waiting times: database study, *British Medical Journal*, 315(7103): 290–2.

Dowling, B. (1998) Potential biases do not affect results of waiting time study, *British Medical Journal*, 317(7150): 79.

Dowling, B. (2000) *GPs and Purchasing in the NHS: The Internal Market and Beyond*. Aldershot: Ashgate.

Ennew, C., Feighan, T. and Whynes, D. (1998) Entrepreneurial activity in the public sector: evidence from UK primary care, in P. Taylor-Gooby (ed.) *Choice and Public Policy*. Basingstoke: Macmillan.

Exworthy, M. (2001) Primary care in the UK: understanding the dynamics of devolution, *Health and Social Care in the Community*, 9(5): 266–78.

Exworthy, M. and Berney, L. (2000) *What counts and what works? Evaluating policies to tackle health inequalities*. Paper presented at a seminar on 'Measuring Success:

What Counts is What Works', in the ESRC Research Seminar Series 'New Labour and the Third Way in Public Services', 20 September 2000. Cardiff: Cardiff Business School.

Ferlie, E., Ashburner, L., Fitzgerald, L. and Pettigrew, A. (1996) *The New Public Management in Action*. Oxford: Oxford University Press.

Giddens, A. (1998) *The Third Way: The Renewal of Social Democracy*. Cambridge: Policy Press.

Greer, S. (2001) *Divergence and Devolution*. London: The Nuffield Trust.

Ham, C. (1996) Primary care led purchasing in the NHS: fundholding and other models, in J. Griffin (ed.) *The Future of Primary Care*. London: Office of Health Economics.

Harrison, S. (1998) The politics of evidence-based medicine in the United Kingdom, *Policy and Politics*, 26(1): 15–31.

Harrison, S. (2002) New Labour, modernisation and the medical labour process, *Journal of Social Policy*, 31(3): 465–86.

HM Treasury (2002) *Budget 2002*, downloaded from www.hm-treasury.gov.uk/budget

Jones, T. (2001) Financing the NHS, in P. Merry (ed.) *Wellard's NHS Handbook 2001/02*, 16th edn. Sussex: JMH Publishing.

Klein, R. (1995) *The New Politics of the NHS*. London: Longman.

Klein, R. (2000) From evidence-based medicine to evidence-based policy? *Journal of Health Services Research and Policy*, 5(2): 65–6.

Labour Party (1993) *GP Fundholding: Bad for Your Health*. London: Labour Party Campaigns and Communications Directorate.

Lee, S. and Woodward, R. (2002) Implementing the Third Way: the delivery of public services under the Blair Government, *Public Money and Management*, 22(4): 49–56.

Le Grand, J., Mays, N. and Dixon, J. (1998) The reforms: success or failure or neither, in J. Le Grand, N. Mays and J. Mulligan (eds) *Learning from the NHS Internal Market: A Review of the Evidence*. London: King's Fund.

Mays, N., Goodwin, N., Killoran, A. and Malbon, G. (1998) *Total Purchasing: A Step towards Primary Care Groups*. London: King's Fund.

Newman, J. (2000) Beyond the new public management? Modernising public services, in J. Clarke, S. Gewirtz and E. McLaughlin (eds) *New Managerialism, New Welfare?* London: Sage.

Newman, J. (2001) *Modernising Governance*. London: Sage.

NHS Confederation (2002) *The New GMS Contract – Delivering the Benefits for GPs and Their Patients*. London: NHS Confederation.

NHS Executive (1994) *Developing NHS Purchasing and GP Fundholding*, EL(94)79. Leeds: NHS Executive.

Nutley, S. and Webb, J. (2000) Evidence and the policy process, in H.T.O. Davies, S.M. Nutley and P.C. Smith (eds) *What Works? Evidence-based Policy and Practice in Public Services*. Bristol: Policy Press.

Owen, J.W. (1998) Introduction, in R. Hazell and P. Jervis (eds) *Devolution and Health*, Nuffield Trust Series 3. London: University College and the Nuffield Trust.

Pater, J.E. (1981) *The Making of the National Health Service*. London: King Edward's Hospital Fund for London.

Paton, C. (2002) New Labour's record on the NHS, in M. Powell (ed.) *Evaluating New Labour's Welfare Reforms*. Bristol: Policy Press.

Pollitt, C. (1995) Justification by works or by faith?, *Evaluation*, 1(2): 133–54.

Powell, M. (ed.) (2002) Introduction, in M. Powell (ed.) *Evaluating New Labour's Welfare Reforms*. Bristol: Policy Press.

Regen, E., Smith, J. and Shapiro, J. (1998) *First off the Starting Block: Lessons from GP Commissioning Pilots for PCGs*. Birmingham: Health Services Management Centre.

Robinson, R. and Le Grand, J. (eds) (1994) *Evaluating the NHS Reforms*. London: King's Fund.

Rouse, J. and Smith, G. (2002) Evaluating New Labour's accountability reforms, in M. Powell (ed.) *Evaluating New Labour's Welfare Reforms*. Bristol: Policy Press.

Rummery, K. (1998) Changes in primary health care policy: the implications for joint commissioning with social services, *Health and Social Care in the Community*, 6(6): 429–37.

Secretary of State for Health (1997) *The New NHS: Modern, Dependable* London: The Stationery Office.

Secretary of State for Health (2000) *The NHS Plan: A Plan for Investment, A Plan for Reform*. London: The Stationery Office.

Secretary of State for Health (2002) *Delivering the NHS Plan: Next Steps on Investment, Next Steps on Reform*. London: The Stationery Office.

Secretary of State for Northern Ireland (1998) *Fit for the Future: A Consultation Document on the Government's Proposals for the Future of Health and Personal Social Services in Northern Ireland*. Belfast: The Stationery Office.

Secretary of State for Scotland (1998) *Designed to Care: Renewing the National Health Service in Scotland*. Edinburgh: The Stationery Office.

Secretary of State for Wales (1998) *NHS Wales: Putting Patients First*, Cardiff: The Stationery Office.

Wilkin, D., Gillam, S. and Leese, B. (eds) (1999) *The National Tracker Survey of Primary Care Groups and Trusts: Progress and Challenges 1999/2000*. Manchester: University of Manchester/London: King's Fund.

Wilkin, D., Gillam, S. and Coleman, A. (eds) (2001) *The National Tracker Survey of Primary Care Groups and Trusts 2000/2001: Modernising the NHS?* Manchester: University of Manchester/London: King's Fund.

Wilkin, D., Coleman, A., Dowling, B. and Smith, K. (2002) *The National Tracker Survey of Primary Care Groups and Trusts 2001/2002: Taking Responsibility?* Manchester: The University of Manchester.

2   Primary care organizations and the 'modernization' of the NHS

Matthew Bond and Julian Le Grand

Introduction

In the White Paper *The New NHS: Modern, Dependable* the Labour government committed itself to finding a 'Third Way' for the National Health
Service (NHS). On the one hand, the new NHS would be steered clear of the
'old centralized command and control system of the 1970s' because it
'stifled innovation and put the needs of institutions ahead of the needs of
patients' (Secretary of State for Health 1997: 10). On the other hand, Labour
did not wish to continue the internal market that had been developed by
the Conservative governments that immediately preceded it, because this
'fragment[ed] decision-making and distort[ed] incentives to such an extent
that unfairness and bureaucracy became its defining features' (Secretary
of State for Health 1997: 10). The specific proposals contained in the
White Paper reflect the wider philosophy of New Labour. This philosophy
attempted to meld features of neo-liberal political thinking, such as
decentralization and close attention to the efficiency of policy initiatives,
with socialist or social democratic ideals, such as equity and fairness. Rather
than limiting policy thinking with allegedly outdated notions of ideological
purity, the aim was to develop a 'Third Way' (Giddens 1998) that moved
'beyond left and right' and where policy considerations would be guided by
what works.

Attempts to bridge the divides that have separated left and right political
philosophies did not start with New Labour. For example, market socialism
(Le Grand and Estrin 1989) attempts to combine public ownership (an
approach typically associated with the left) with market mechanisms (an
approach typically associated with the right). Quasi-markets in publicly supplied services resemble the approach described by market socialists. Another
example is the failed Clinton health plan of the 1990s in the USA. This
intended to employ public and private funding in a health system that would
also use competition between providers to supply health services to patients,

Table 2.1 Ownership and governance dimensions and their ideological connotations

	Ownership	*Governance*
Socialist/social democratic	public	hierarchical
Neo-liberal	private	market
Market socialist	public	market
Third Way	public/private hybrids	market/hierarchical hybrids

who would be represented by health alliances made up of large corporate purchasers of health care. Such approaches combine the two separate dimensions of ownership (public or private) and governance (market or hierarchical) in untraditional ways. They treat the two dimensions as orthogonal, in that they can be combined in ways that vary with the aims of the implementers of policy. (Whether this is true is beyond the scope of this paper, but see De Jasay (1990) for a neo-Liberal critique.) Table 2.1 shows the two dimensions, together with their ideological connotations.

The Labour government has adopted a slightly different approach. Rather than trying to combine the two dimensions in novel ways, the government has instead tried to move beyond simple public/private and hierarchy/market dichotomies. The Third Way treats each of these dimensions as a continuum and has developed policy initiatives that sit between or, to use a bolder characterization, transcend the extreme positions of the continuum. An example of the government's mixing of public and private ownership is the use of the Private Finance Initiative to fund the building of new NHS hospitals. Initiatives like these are attracting increasing controversy and are prevalent in education, transport and the funding of public service infrastructure. However, their impact on primary care has so far been limited (although there are increasing signs that their impact will grow); instead, policy developments in primary care have tended to involve the blending of hierarchical and market mechanisms.

Our aim in this chapter is to explore the consequences for primary care of this approach. We do so by first placing the primary care reforms in the context of wider policy developments in the NHS (Bartlett and Le Grand 1993). We then develop an analytical framework for assisting in the evaluation of primary care groups and trusts (PCG/Ts) which is akin to the quasi-market framework that was developed to evaluate performance in the internal market. We conclude by looking to what the future of PCG/Ts might hold. In discussing the successes and limitations of these new organizations, the characteristics of Third Way organizations in general, which attempt to blend hierarchical and market mechanisms, will be illustrated.

The institutional development of primary care groups/trusts

Precedents in the internal market

The central policy innovation of the internal market that affected primary care was the devolution of some commissioning budgets, practice infrastructure budgets and prescribing budgets to 'fundholding' general practices. The intention of this policy was to combine the special knowledge that general practitioners (GPs) had of both their patients and local providers of acute services with the incentives of managing a cash-limited budget to commission services efficiently. Although fundholding was based on a model of individual choice and market mechanisms of coordination, it prompted the development, by GPs and others working in primary care, of new primary care organizations. These organizations ranged from locality commissioning groups, where groups of GPs advised health authorities but did not assume budgetary responsibilities, to total purchasing pilots, where groups of general practices were granted powers to assume full responsibility (although none actually did) for the full range of hospital and community health services, as well as retaining the other budgetary responsibilities of ordinary GP fundholders.

What united all these organizational developments was the involvement of GPs in planning local health services. In the light of GPs' history as independent contractors in the NHS, characterized by a lack of cooperation with each other and a lack of involvement in planning and managing health services, these organizations represented a major step in the development of primary care. Ironically, given the fact that the internal market was so heavily underpinned by principles of individual choice and was criticized for 'fragmenting' the health service, it nevertheless witnessed the development of multi-practice groups involved in collectively planning health services for their patients.

The New NHS and primary care organizations

Rather than entirely eschewing these developments, the Labour government built on and extended them. Fundholding was abolished and all general practices were compelled to become members of a primary care group (PCG) – subsequently primary care trusts (PCTs). However, the purchaser–provider split was retained. Primary care organizations, in which GPs were still strongly represented, would therefore retain responsibility for purchasing, or commissioning as it has since been renamed (see Light 1998; also Chapter 9), hospital and community health care services. The greatest difference was that *all* GPs would now be represented by commissioning organizations which resembled the collective commissioning organizations, such as total purchasing pilots, that developed during the internal market. It was no longer possible for individual GP practices to commission or purchase acute services, or to remain entirely outside of any primary care commissioning organization (as had non-fundholding GPs who had not belonged to any locality commissioning group).

The Labour government's reforms therefore not only accelerated trends towards collective commissioning that had begun during the internal market, they also extended the scope of primary care organizations' responsibilities. As well as commissioning acute services, PCG/Ts were now also charged with new responsibilities for public health and for clinical governance; primary care organizations would become responsible for the prevention of disease and for the quality of services provided by their GP practices. Although total purchasing pilots and locality commissioning groups had devoted some attention to these issues, the creation of PCG/Ts ensured that they would be central functions of primary care in New Labour's NHS. Thus while its role during the internal market had been to modernize and increase efficiency in secondary care through the effective purchasing and commissioning of services, primary care was now also charged with responsibility for modernizing itself. Finally, PCG/Ts extended the representation of interests within primary care organizations. While locality commissioning groups and total purchasing pilots had been led and organized largely by GPs, PCG/Ts explicitly include a broader range of primary care interests. Practice and community nurses, local authority social services department representatives and lay representatives were included on PCG boards and this broader representation has been maintained with the transition to PCTs. Although GPs were dominant on the boards of PCGs, their role has been reduced in PCTs, where the influence of non-executives and other primary care professionals is much greater.

In summary, although the proposals in *The New NHS* built on organizational forms that developed during the internal market, they also introduced several important changes. These changes were the inclusion of all GPs in PCG/Ts, the extension of primary care organizations' responsibilities to include public health and quality issues, and the representation of a wide range of primary care interests in PCG/Ts. The planning and management roles that primary care services had begun to assume during the internal market were intensified, as actors who previously had had only a minimal role in NHS decision-making were brought into the centre of the new primary care organizations.

Organizational principles of primary care groups/trusts

At the time of their creation, it would have been difficult to be optimistic about the prospects for PCG/Ts in successfully adopting the roles expected of them in

The New NHS. Their closest organizational precedent, total purchasing pilots, had faced some major challenges. Despite some significant successes, total purchasing pilots had difficulty assuming responsibility for much of their commissioning budgets; they were more successful in changing services at the primary–secondary interface rather than within secondary care proper; and they had difficulties in changing the behaviour of their member GPs and practices (Le Grand *et al.* 1998). It should also be noted that because membership of total purchasing pilots was voluntary, it is likely that those practices most likely to succeed had actually joined the scheme. Having an organizational precedent with such a mixed record, there was little guarantee that PCG/Ts, with their greater responsibilities, could exceed the achievements of total purchasing pilots. Beyond providing a forum for primary care interests to express themselves, and expanding their range of primary care responsibilities, what social mechanisms were available to PCG/Ts to ensure that they formed a cohesive identity and exert control over their members?

Local responsibility and cooperation

Two principles of organizational management are repeated throughout the major policy documents relating to *The New NHS* in general and to primary care in particular. The first is the devolution of responsibility to lower levels, rather than keeping power at the centre. One of the six principles of *The New NHS*, as listed in the White Paper, was 'local responsibility'. The White Paper also claimed that 'For the first time in the history of the NHS all the primary care professionals, who do the majority of prescribing, treating and referring will have control over how resources are best used to benefit patients' (Secretary of State for Health 1997: 37). This commitment to local responsibility has recently been reiterated in *Delivering the NHS Plan*, which restated the need to 'devolve decisions to frontline staff' (Secretary of State for Health 2002: 9) and to 'reduce hierarchies and develop self-managed teams' (p. 25). Whether local responsibility is compatible with the development of national standards such as national service frameworks, and national regulatory bodies such as the Commission for Health Improvement and its successor the Commission for Health Care Audit and Inspection, is a question that will be developed later in this chapter. At this point, it is necessary only to assert that one of the organizational principles underpinning the creation of PCG/Ts was local responsibility and the devolution of power.

The other important principle underpinning the Labour government's approach to the NHS was a rejection of the competitive and conflictual relations that developed during the internal market. Cooperation and partnership were to be the coordinating mechanisms that would replace both command and control and competition (see also Chapters 9 and 12). The 1997 White

Paper claimed that the 'Third Way' approach to managing the NHS was 'based on partnership' and partnership was one of the White Paper's six principles. Rather than competing in markets or taking orders from central agencies, it was claimed that actors in the NHS should find their common interests and promote these through cooperative mechanisms.

How did these general organizational aims manifest themselves? What institutional mechanisms were available to ensure these aims would influence the actions of members of the new primary care organizations? So far as local responsibility is concerned, the mechanism by which this principle was to be implemented was the involvement of local primary care actors on important decision-making committees in PCG/Ts, including the PCG board, the PCT executive committee and subgroups dealing with specific PCG/T functions. At board level local actors have an opportunity to review the organization's policies, whereas at executive committee level and subgroup levels they have the opportunity to formulate those policies. Through subcommittees dealing with topics ranging from clinical governance to prescribing, a wide variety of local health professionals have been granted a substantial formal role in primary care decision-making.

What mechanisms are available to guarantee the operation of the second organizational principle, that of cooperation? Apart from relying purely on GPs' latent professionalism, a likely candidate is the unified budget now held by PCG/Ts. As Majeed and Malcolm (1999) have pointed out, 'resource decisions taken by one practice in a Primary Care Group will impact directly on others' (p. 772). How does this occur? The unified budget permits transfers between three budgets that had previously been kept separate – those for prescribing, hospital and community health services and the cash-limited general medical services budget that funds practice infrastructure. To allay the fears of GPs that practice infrastructure funds might be siphoned off to pay for overspends on prescribing or hospital and community health services, resources can only be diverted from the cash-limited general medical services budget with the consent of local GPs. In exchange for this, cash-limited infrastructure funds are only permitted to grow at the rate of inflation, wheras the other two budget headings can show real (greater than inflation) growth. This arrangement has the consequence that the size of the cash-limited general medical services infrastructure budget that benefits GPs most in their roles as individual, independent contractors will be determined by the referral and prescribing patterns of all GPs in a PCG/T.

However, this arrangement does not necessarily require cooperation between the GPs within a PCG/T. The 1997 White Paper stated that:

> ... over time, the Government expects that Groups will extend indicative budgets to individual practices for the full range of services ... It will be open to the Group to agree practice-level incentive

arrangements associated with these budgets . . . Initially, every practice will have a prescribing budget, as most do now.
(Secretary of State for Health 1997: 38)

Indeed, the creation of indicative budgets potentially replicates the mechanisms used under the fundholding regime to control GPs' expenditure-related
behaviours, because it devolves to individual practices responsibility and
incentives for maintaining budgetary control. Although this option was part
of the government's proposed reforms, its realization has been limited. For
example, in the second round of the Tracker Survey of PCG/Ts, only 6 per cent
of PCG/Ts reported that their practices held devolved budgets for hospital and
community health services budgets and only two of seventy-one PCG/Ts had
attached incentives to these; two-thirds had financial incentive schemes
linked to their prescribing budgets; and approximately half had or planned to
attach financial incentive schemes to clinical governance targets (Wilkin *et al.*
2001). Therefore, in the absence of devolved, practice-level budgets, cooperative mechanisms must be relied upon to facilitate efficient use of resources by
general practices. As Majeed and Malcolm (1999) state, 'To manage their unified budgets effectively, general practitioners will have to work collaboratively
with other practices in their group' (p. 772). However, this still begs the question of what cooperative or collaborative mechanisms they can and will use. It
is still far from clear that a Third Way has emerged in primary care that can
blend hierarchical and market mechanisms without suffering from the failures
that are associated with them.

Community governance

How should one characterize PCG/Ts organizationally? One possibility is
to conceptualize them as network organizations (Powell 1990) that rely on
consensus and upon horizontal, rather than vertical, chains of command.
However, while this term reflects the semi-formal nature of the identity and
governance of these organizations, it fails to capture other features, such as the
importance of democracy, professional leadership and inter-professional trust,
that will be important features of PCG/Ts if the inclusive nature of collective
decision-making is to be successful. Although the importance of networks is
not doubted, it is likely that many GPs have few links with other GPs within the
PCG/T, compared to the quantity and quality of the ties they have with central
government. Another term that has been used as an alternative to markets and
hierarchies is 'community' (Lichbach 1995; Posner 2000). This allows a simul-
taneous focus on issues of corporate identity and on the ways in which PCG/Ts
control their members and guide them towards desired ends. It also connects
the discussion to concepts that have been used by scholars, ranging from
Etzioni (1993) to Putman (2000), who have influenced Third Way thinking.

For the purposes of this chapter, community governance can be described as a system of governance where the rights to control behaviour are decentralized to individual health professionals, but where the consequences of their behaviours are felt by health professionals collectively. The community may consist of all those health professionals who feel the consequences of each other's behaviours, or a subset of health professionals who are, more or less, arbitrarily mandated by the state to act as a community. Technically speaking, within this conceptual framework communities are determined by a combination of externalities and state prescription. This definition contrasts with market-based systems, where individual actors have the right to control behaviour but are the only ones to feel the consequences of that behaviour, and hierarchically based systems, where a central actor has both rights of control over the behaviour of other actors and the right to distribute the benefits of that behaviour as he or she wishes. The salience of this definition arises from the fact that, to date, the reforms to the NHS have not explicitly encroached on GPs' clinical freedoms, nor have they greatly threatened their independent contractor status – although, as Majeed and Malcolm (1999) point out, the reforms have increased GPs' dependency on each other. As Table 2.1 showed, this structure of intra-organizational dependencies represents a Third Way that blends elements of hierarchy and market.

How does the concept of community governance assist in the analysis and evaluation of PCG/Ts? In what follows, the same model of a rational utility-maximizing actor that was used in, for instance, Bartlett and Le Grand's (1993) model of quasi-markets will be employed to explore the community properties of PCG/Ts. The model assumes that the actors remain the same, whether they are in a community, hierarchy or market; rather, it is only the institutional environment that changes. While sociologists might criticize this assumption for its naivety, it is part of a trade-off between realism and analytic power. To the extent, therefore, that the assumption is true, the analysis will add insights to the mechanisms guiding PCG/Ts.

A further potential problem with this approach is that the concept of community governance is often associated with notions of trust, leadership, social norms and networks. For example, Scally and Donaldson (1999), in their discussion of clinical governance, argue that leadership and culture are important elements of a successful clinical governance strategy, because it depends on decentralized and informal mechanisms of governance. These notions are not readily associated with rational actors and the associated theory of choice, as they are thought to be incompatible with the model of self-interested actors that characterizes rational choice analyses. Instead, they are linked more closely to models of actors motivated by meaning or ritual; indeed, it could be claimed that they are beyond the scope of rational actor models. However, scholars in sociology (e.g. Gambetta 1993), political science (e.g. Chong 1991), economics (e.g. Chwe 2001) and game theory (Kreps and Wilson 1982) are increasingly using rational actor models to explain behaviours and social outcomes that were previously associated with irrational motives. Some central implications of these approaches will be used in the next section to highlight important dimensions of PCG/Ts.

The effect of community governance on the effectiveness of primary care groups/trusts

Unlike Bartlett and Le Grand (1993), who were able to draw on a comprehensive and unified body of research in their exploration of quasi-markets, research on the concept of community governance is scattered across many disciplines and often has quite different objectives. There is no single, rational choice theory of community governance. To facilitate discussion and highlight some important features of the organization of PCG/Ts, two common examples of social behaviour in PCG/Ts will be discussed. These examples have been selected to draw attention to the ability of PCG/Ts to achieve their objectives. This analysis is far from complete, but provides the point for further debate on the organizational features of PCG/Ts.

Example 1

Research into decision-making at board level (Smith *et al.* 2001) has found that PCG/Ts have acute difficulty achieving corporacy; that is, the board has difficulty reaching a common view, with different interests – especially those represented by GPs – pursuing minority, sectional aims.

Should the lack of corporacy achieved by PCG/T boards come as a surprise? Do difficulties of corporacy arise because many primary care actors, especially GPs, are not used to participating in corporate decision-making? Will consensus develop over time, as GPs and other board members gain experience of collective decision-making, or are these problems more intractable? How can the organizational principle of local responsibility be sustained if local actors cannot reach a common viewpoint? A hypothetical example might provide an answer to these questions.

Table 2.2 shows an example of a hypothetical collective decision-making problem. It shows the different preferences of three GPs for three different clinics to which patients could be referred for a routine problem. To explore the difficulties of arriving at a collective decision, in this example it is useful to see what would happen if the participants attempted to reach a collective decision using majority-rule, pairwise voting. This is a common method of arriving at collective decisions and involves first voting on two alternatives; the winner then goes on to face another alternative, until there is only one alternative remaining. If majority-rule, pairwise voting is used, then clinic 1

Table 2.2 A hypothetical example of a collective decision-making problem: GPs' preferences for three clinics

	Clinic 1	Clinic 2	Clinic 3
GP A	1*	2	3
GP B	3	1	2
GP C	2	3	1

* These numbers represent the preferences of each GP for each clinic. For example, GP A's most preferred option is clinic 1, her second is clinic 2 and her least preferred option is clinic 3.

would be preferred over clinic 2 because GPs A and C prefer clinic 1 to clinic 2. Clinic 2 would be preferred over clinic 3 because GPs A and B prefer 2 to 3. Clinic 3 would be preferred to clinic 1 because GPs B and C prefer 3 to 1. Using this method, each alternative is able to garner a majority against one of the other alternatives. This leads to an outcome where collective preferences create a cycle in which 1 defeats 2 defeats 3 defeats 1 and so on. No consistent decision is possible.

This result is not simply a consequence of the way the example is structured. Under some modes of structuring individual preferences, it is true that inconsistencies would not result and collective preferences would have some meaning; in other words, if the GPs in the example valued the clinics differently, then inconsistencies would not occur. However, as the number of decision-makers and the number of choices increase, then the proportion of possible individual preferences that lead to inconsistent collective preferences also increases. The more complex the decision is, the more likely that inconsistent and incoherent collective preferences will result. As the delivery of health care is highly complex, with many possible dimensions to consider, these difficulties are likely to loom large for PCG/T decision-making.

This is not simply the result either of using majority-rule, pairwise voting as a heuristic device to explore the difficulties of determining collective preferences; these difficulties are attached to all methods of arriving at collective decisions. Arrow's (1963) possibility theorem has shown that there is no collective decision-making process that does not violate a minimal set of desirable democratic criteria. No matter what institutional guise the process takes, it will be vulnerable to problems like inconsistent collective preferences. Alternatively, collective decision-making processes will inevitably violate certain basic democratic desiderata, for example, by not allowing all actors to have a say in the decision because of their incompatible individual preferences or by relying on a 'dictator' to make decisions for the collective. Although dictatorship and democracy carry strong normative connotations, the underlying issue is whether the decision-making powers available to the collective consists of a set of individuals with each individual having as much influence as all others; or whether there is a single actor within the collective who is granted ultimate decision-making powers.

In reality, collectives are constantly making decisions; they are not hampered by the difficulties that have been highlighted in this discussion. However, this does not get around the fact that, unless by remarkable coincidence these collectives have not faced any situations where there are inconsistencies in collective decision-making, some actors are exercising 'dictatorial' powers. There is the danger that a lack of formal decision-making processes in PCG/Ts obscures the fact that some actors are acting as dictators. Rather than trying to avoid 'dictatorial' decision-making, which is probably impossible in the complex environments characterizing healthcare delivery, there are several possible institutional mechanisms available to PCG/Ts that can mitigate these problems. Institutional mechanisms can lead individual decision-makers towards collective decisions, even if their individual preferences do not point obviously to collective decisions (Riker 1982), so it is important to be aware of possible institutional influences and how these relate to the aims of PCG/Ts. Some possibilities are listed below.

Primary care group/trust boards and executive committees as consultative bodies
Although collective decisions may ultimately be dictatorial, the inclusion of multiple interests on boards and executive committees can have a consultative function that is consistent with the spirit of democratic decision-making. For instance, the inclusion of multiple interests can eliminate unanimously unpopular decisions. Looking at the example shown in Table 2.2, a fourth clinic could be added. All three GPs might have unanimously rejected this clinic because it was run by a specialist who was particularly disliked by the GPs' patients. If that information was only available to GPs by virtue of their close relationship with their patients, then their unanimous rejection of clinic 4 would prevent it being selected by a 'dictator' who did not have access to this information.

The difficulty with this mechanism is that it gives PCG/T stakeholders an incentive to obfuscate and conceal their interests; interested parties are unlikely to provide impartial or entirely honest advice (Milgrom and Roberts 1987, 1990). Decisions based on consultation with interested parties, such as decisions made by PCG/T boards that rely on advice from GPs, may be suboptimal because they are based on biased information. Such decisions are also likely to lead to unproductive efforts at lobbying, if GPs devote time to influencing the decisions of PCG/T boards instead of supplying healthcare to their patients. Because PCG/Ts have probably introduced the greatest changes for GPs, compared with other primary care interests, it should not be surprising if they devote more energy than any other interest represented on PCG/T boards to influencing PCG/T politics.

Division of dictatorial powers

Perhaps the central normative objection to dictatorship is the unfairness associated with concentrating so much power in the hands of a single individual or group of individuals. One way of overcoming this problem is to divide dictatorial power. Dividing complex decisions into separate components allows them to become more soluble (Shepsle 1979), as well as allowing different interests to act as dictators. This can be achieved by rotating or delegating dictatorial powers across different stakeholders. The proliferation of subgroups and committees in PCG/Ts might be explained by the desire to divide dictatorial powers. This leads to an expectation that those PCG/Ts with especially diverse interests, and hence the greatest difficulty in arriving at rational collective preferences, will be likely to have more subgroups. Subgroups become efficient mechanisms for reaching decisions, as they offer ways of resolving difficult political disputes among actors in PCG/Ts.

The importance of culture

Cultural factors are repeatedly cited as important influences on the ability of health professionals to deliver successfully on NHS objectives, especially by observers concerned with the implementation of clinical governance (Scally and Donaldson 1999; Marshall *et al.* 2002). Why is this? One possibility is that inconsistent collective preferences occur when actors base their judgements on diverse dimensions or facets of the same problem. Looking again at the example of selecting a clinic (Table 2.2), if the three actors are focusing on different aspects of the clinic and weighting these differently, then inconsistent preferences are more likely. If their judgements are based only on the same, single dimension, such as some notion of equity, then inconsistencies will not occur (Black 1948). As Riker (1982) has argued, 'If, by reason of discussion, debate, civic education, and political socialization, voters have a common view of the political dimension . . . then a transitive [i.e. consistent] outcome is guaranteed' (p. 128). One would expect that less diverse PCG/Ts would have less difficulty determining collective preferences. The importance of culture also highlights the importance of leadership in inculcating a common purpose among the different members of PCG/Ts.

National targets as dictator

Perhaps the most drastic solution to the problem is to cede local decision-making powers altogether to central government. Despite the emphasis that has been placed on devolved local responsibility in official government documents, central government has increasingly assumed agenda-setting powers through measures such as the national service frameworks. While lending coherence to PCG/T decision-making, this nevertheless also undermines attempts to devolve decision-making responsibilities to local actors.

Summary of the main difficulties with collective decision-making
The central issue that this discussion has highlighted is that, as decisions become more complex, so democratic decision-making processes become less coherent. When faced with the complex environment of health care delivery, minimal democratic criteria will inevitably have to be sacrificed if decisions are to be made. Each of the four mechanisms discussed above reduce problems of irrational collective preferences and the difficulties that these cause for democratic decision-making; however, in each case this is only achieved through the loss of some influence by the collective. The discussion has also shown why community decision-making might have undemocratic connotations – democratic decisions can also be inefficient and incoherent decisions.

Example 2

We have conducted a study of seven PCG/Ts in London and eastern England. This has involved interviewing all board and executive committee members and conducting surveys of health professionals who are non-board/executive committee members. The study aimed to explore the effects of PCG/Ts' organizational structures on the types of decisions they make and on their ability to implement those decisions. One of the questions that we asked board and executive committee members is whether PCG/Ts could have coped without having GP chairs of boards or executive committees or without having GP members altogether. We wished to discover whether decisions that have been taken and implemented could have been taken if GPs had been absent from PCG/Ts. Almost without exception the response has been that the implementation of decisions has depended on the presence of GPs in positions of decision-making responsibility. This response has not been restricted to GPs.

Why does the presence of GPs legitimate decisions that would otherwise not have been possible? The answer probably lies in the fact that GP board and executive committee members can gain the trust of their colleagues where bureaucrats could not. However, this still begs the question as to what factors induce GPs to trust each other and distrust bureaucrats. By modelling the situation, the specific factors that induce trust can be clarified. Modelling situations involving trust also demonstrates the general difficulty that social dilemmas create for community organizations. Social dilemmas occur when all actors make rational choices but the aggregate result is irrational, in the sense that another result is technically possible but socially inaccessible, given the preferences of the individual actors. The development of trust provides an important mechanism for overcoming social dilemmas.

Figure 2.1 displays a trust game (Dasgupta 1988; Kreps 1990; Buskens 1998). It shows the case where a trustor (the person placing trust) must decide whether to place trust in a trustee (the person receiving trust). The trustor faces

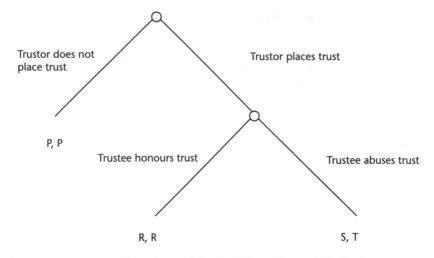

Figure 2.1 Trust game. Trustor's payoff: R > P > S; Trustee's payoff: T > R > P.

a dilemma. If s/he places trust, then the trustee has an incentive to violate that trust to acquire a short-term gain (S, T). The trustor looking at this situation will not place trust because s/he does not want to risk being tricked by the trustee (P, P). If the trustor does not place trust, then each receives a payoff lower than another possible payoff that each *could* receive if the trustor placed trust that was honoured (R, R). This example simultaneously demonstrates both the risk of placing trust and the cost of mistrust.

What can this abstract model tell us about trust in PCG/Ts? There are several similarities between this model and attempts to implement changes relating to clinical governance and other quality initiatives. While a GP might want to improve the quality of her practice, s/he might not want to give the PCG/T relevant information because it could be used against him/her. For example, the GP might fear a reduction in any budgets s/he receives, or might fear a loss of status if his/her practice is revealed to be less efficient than others. Before revealing information, the GP will want to know that it will not be used against him/her. The PCG/T will want the information so that it can improve the quality of medical care provided by its practitioners. However, the PCG/T has the option of penalizing GPs that reveal poor quality by, for example, reducing practice investment or using the practice as an example to others of bad practice. The PCG/T, therefore, needs a way of signalling (Posner 2000) that it can be trusted and will not succumb to the temptation of violating the trust that has been placed in it.

How can this challenge be overcome? One solution is suggested by the theory of repeated games. If both sides know that they are likely to play this game an indefinite number of times, then there is a greater chance that the trustor will place trust with the trustee than in the case of a single play. Why? The reason is simply that, by abusing the trust placed in him, the trustee may never have trust placed in him again. The trustee must balance the short-term gains derived from violating trust against the long-term value of the relationship. The more that the trustee values the future or expects to interact with the trustor, the more likely s/he is to honour the trust placed in him/her.

To make this model relevant to the example that we are focusing on, it is useful to examine the ability of trustors to determine whether trustees are likely to honour trust because they want the relationship to continue. This will depend both on the way the trustee discounts future payoffs and the likelihood that the trustor and trustee will meet again (Bendor and Mookherjee 1987). Applying this model to the example of PCG/Ts and GPs, the trustors can be thought of as GPs and the trustees can be thought of as the PCG/T. General practitioners will need to infer the value that PCG/Ts place on continuing the relationship; in other words, they have to infer the trustworthiness of the PCG/Ts. The model points to several factors that will promote the placing of trust by GPs in the PCG/T:

- *The importance of the long term.* When determining the trustworthiness of the PCG/T, a GP will be more likely to attribute trustworthiness if s/he feels that the members of the PCG/T s/he is dealing with will be around in the long term. A trustee who is likely to move on has a greater incentive to violate trust. For example, a GP might feel that a manager would like to be able to state on his CV that s/he has 'sorted out' the PCG/T before moving on to another posting. The mobility of the trustee is likely to induce less trust in the trustor GP. The value of having a fellow GP in the role of trustee immediately becomes apparent. General practitioners are less mobile than managers, as their status as independent contractor means that they have a financial investment in a geographically rooted practice. This also implies that salaried GPs who enjoy greater job mobility might be less successful in the role of trustee. It also reflects the common disdain with which interviewees in our study displayed towards the idea of public health doctors replacing GPs on PCG/T boards. The important dimension is not so much based on intra-professional likes and dislikes, as having a long-term future in the community.

  Another factor affecting a GP's perception of the trustworthiness of a PCG/T is the extent to which national policies are subject to change (Hausmann and Le Grand 1999). The model predicts that if the GP feels that the PCG/T is not committed to the long-term basis of the relationship then s/he will perceive it as less trustworthy. A stable policy environment should allow levels of perceived trustworthiness to rise. A manager working in a stable policy environment will therefore be perceived as more trustworthy than a manager working in a constantly changing policy environment.

• *The importance of repeated interaction.* Even if GPs feel that PCG/T managers place a relatively high value on future interactions, this will not mean as much if they feel that future interactions are unlikely. This is another advantage that local GPs have in the role of trustee over other potential candidates for the role; they are embedded (Granovetter 1985) in the local community of GPs, so they are likely to have a greater number of inter-actions with potential trustees. The trust game is nested (Tsebelis 1990) in multiple games with other GPs, so they have more to lose by violating trust in one setting.

• *The importance of culture.* Game theory has shown that, although trust can be maintained if interaction is repeated, there are multiple ways in which trust can be maintained between PCG/Ts and GPs (Schelling 1960; Kreps 1990; Miller 1992). For example, some GPs may have stronger cultures of trust, which will allow them to accept certain violations of trust compared with others. Primary care groups and trusts with different cultures will have stronger or weaker trust-based cooperative relationships as a consequence (Chwe 2001). The difficulty is that culture is not so malleable and again depends on long-term investment.

These two examples show that PCG/Ts can forge corporate identities that take collective decisions and implement those decisions, but this ability depends on certain key variables. In terms of collective identity, it is helpful if the organization's members attach similar values to the different dimensions underlying collective decisions, or have developed mechanisms for mitigating the dangers of dictatorship associated with collective decision-making. In terms of achieving collective action, policy stability is important, as are long-term commitments and strategies on the part of the actors who implement the decisions of PCG/Ts. Ultimately, however, the potential failures of markets and hierarchies are only replaced by the potential failures of community organizations. There is no risk-free road to the implementation of primary care reforms.

Conclusions

There is mounting evidence that PCG/Ts are not any more successful than the primary care organizations that preceded them. In relation to the commission-ing of services, they appear to have made little progress (Bond 2002) or appear ill-placed to accept the commissioning responsibilities that lie before them (Baxter *et al.* 2002; see also Chapter 9). The earlier experiences of total purchas-ing pilots suggest that these difficulties are not unexpected. In summary, PCG/

Ts are likely to experience difficulties for one or more of the following reasons. First, PCG/Ts may find it hard to deal with organizational failures such as irrational collective preferences or lack of trust. Their preoccupation with organizational matters in their first 2 years of existence are evidence of this possibility. Secondly, the principle of local responsibility may be at odds with the principle of re-establishing a 'national' health service. The strong national pressures to 'modernize' the NHS may undermine local initiatives. For example, new national targets could drive down GPs' estimates of the trustworthiness of PCG/Ts. Thirdly, it is possible that the present state of primary care, whether by intention or by accident, is only another step on the way to consolidating trends that were set in motion during the internal market, of bringing GPs into a 'managed NHS'. Alongside the creation of community organizations there has been experimentation with more hierarchical coordinating mechanisms. Personal medical service pilot schemes, for example, have experimented with local contracts that are made between PCG/Ts and general practices, which allow for services to be tailored to specific local circumstances. Personal medical service pilot schemes have also facilitated the expansion of salaried general practice. These trends may be further accelerated by plans for the new GP contract (see Chapter 1 for further details of both personal medical services and the proposed new GP contract). The replacement of GPs as independent contractors with GPs as salaried employees will mean a long-term trend towards a much more hierarchically controlled primary care sector.

In 1998, Klein and Maynard wrote about the creation of PCG/Ts:

> The attractions for government of creating a situation in which general practitioners improve resource use by controlling their colleagues are self-evident. The attractions for independent contractor general practitioners are less apparent and they may not comply. Indeed, the long-term implication may be that ministers expect general practitioners to become salaried employees.
>
> (Klein and Maynard 1998: 5)

Their statement is becoming increasingly prophetic. Regardless of whether PCG/Ts are cracking under their own contradictions, under the pressures of national standards or whether they are merely a transitional step on the way to a fully managed primary care service, it is becoming increasingly apparent that the 'Third Way' of organizing primary care is not without difficulties. It is unclear whether the modernization of the NHS will be delivered through present structures. Rather than finding a 'Third Way' that blends the best of market and hierarchy, there is a danger that the new primary care organizations will combine the anarchy of market relations with the dictatorship of hierarchy.

References

Arrow, K. (1963) *Social Choice and Individual Values*. London: Wiley.

Bartlett, W. and Le Grand, J. (1993) The theory of quasi-markets, in J. Le Grand and W. Bartlett (eds) *Quasi-markets and Social Policy*. London: Macmillan.

Baxter, K., Shepherd, J., Weiss, M. and Le Grand, J. (2002) Ready steady stop, *Health Service Journal*, 112(5796): 28–9.

Bendor, J. and Mookherjee, D. (1987) Institutional structure and the logic of ongoing collective action, *American Political Science Review*, 81(1): 129–54.

Black, D. (1948) On the rationale of group decision making, *Journal of Political Economy*, 16(1): 23–34.

Bond, M. (2002) Nurture not nature, *Health Service Journal*, 112(5793): 30–1.

Buskens, V. (1998) The social structure of trust, *Social Networks*, 20(3): 265–98.

Chong, D. (1991) *Collective Action and the Civil Rights Movement*. Chicago, IL: University of Chicago Press.

Chwe, M. (2001) *Rational Ritual: Culture, Coordination and Common Knowledge*. Princeton, NJ: Princeton University Press.

Dasgupta, P. (1988) Trust as a commodity, in D. Gambetta (ed.) *Trust: Making and Breaking Cooperative Relations*. Oxford: Blackwell.

De Jasay, A. (1990) *Market Socialism*. London: Institute of Economic Affairs.

Etzioni, A. (1993) *The Spirit of Community: Rights, Responsibilities and the Communitarian Agenda*. New York: Crown Publishers.

Gambetta, D. (1993) *The Sicilian Mafia*. Cambridge, MA: Harvard University Press.

Giddens, A. (1998) *The Third Way: The Renewal of Social Democracy*. Oxford: Policy Press.

Granovetter, M. (1985) Economic action, social structure: the problem of embeddedness, *American Journal of Sociology*, 83(3): 1420–43.

Hausmann, D. and Le Grand, J. (1999) Incentives and health policy: primary and secondary care in the British National Health Service, *Social Science and Medicine*, 49(10): 1299–1307.

Klein, R. and Maynard, A. (1998) On the way to Calvary, *British Medical Journal*, 317(7150): 5.

Kreps, D. (1990) *A Course in Microeconomic Theory*. London: Harvester Wheatsheaf.

Kreps, D. and Wilson, R. (1982) Reputation and imperfect information, *Journal of Economic Theory*, 27(3): 253–79.

Le Grand, J. and Estrin, S. (eds) (1989) *Market Socialism*. Oxford: Clarendon Press.

Le Grand, J., Mays, N. and Mulligan, J. (eds) (1998) *Learning from the NHS Internal Market*. London: King's Fund.

Lichbach, M. (1995) *Rebel's Dilemma*. Ann Arbor, MI: The University of Michigan Press.

Light, D. (1998) *Effective Commissioning: Lessons from Purchasing in American Managed Care*. London: Office of Health Economics.

Majeed, A. and Malcolm, L. (1999) Unified budgets for primary care groups, *British Medical Journal*, 318(7186): 772–6.

Marshall, M., Sheaff, R., Roger, A. *et al.* (2002) A qualitative study of the cultural changes in primary care organisations needed to implement clinical governance, *British Journal of General Practice*, 52(8): 641–5.

Milgrom, P. and Roberts, J. (1987) An economic approach to influence activities and organizational responses, *American Journal of Sociology*, s94: 154–79.

Milgrom, P. and Roberts, J. (1990) Bargaining costs, influence costs and the organization of economic activity, in J. Alt and K. Shepsle (eds) *Perspectives on Positive Political Economy*. Cambridge: Cambridge University Press.

Miller, G. (1992) *Managerial Dilemmas: The Political Economy of Hierarchy.* Cambridge: Cambridge University Press.

Posner, E. (2000) *Law and Social Norms.* Cambridge, MA: Harvard University Press.

Powell, W. (1990) Neither market nor hierarchy: network forms of organization, in L.L. Cummings and B. Shaw (eds) *Research in Organizational Behaviour*, Vol. 12. Greenwich, CT: JAI Press.

Putman, R. (2000) *Bowling Alone: The Collapse and Revival of American Community.* New York: Touchstone.

Riker, W. (1982) *Liberalism against Populism: A Confrontation between the Theory of Democracy and the Theory of Social Choice.* Oxford: Freeman.

Scally, G. and Donaldson, L. (1999) Looking forward: clinical governance and the drive for quality improvement in the NHS in England, *British Medical Journal*, 321(7150): 1559–61.

Schelling, T. (1960) *The Strategy of Conflict.* Cambridge, MA: Harvard University Press.

Secretary of State for Health (1997) *The New NHS: Modern, Dependable.* London: The Stationery Office.

Secretary of State for Health (2002) *Delivering the NHS Plan: Next Steps on Investment, Next Steps on Reform.* London: The Stationery Office.

Shepsle, K. (1979) Institutional arrangements and equilibrium in multidimensional voting models, *American Journal of Political Science*, 68(2): 27–59.

Smith, J., Regen, E., Goodwin, N., McLeod, H. and Shapiro, J. (2001) *Passing on the Baton: Final Report of a National Evaluation of Primary Care Groups and Trusts.* Birmingham: University of Birmingham.

Tsebelis, G. (1990) *Nested Games: Rational Choice in Comparative Politics.* Berkeley, CA: University of California Press.

Wilkin, D., Gillam, S. and Coleman, A. (eds) (2001) *The National Tracker Survey of Primary Care Groups and Trusts 2000/2001: Modernising the NHS?* Manchester: University of Manchester/London: King's Fund.

3 English primary care organizations in an international context

Ray Robinson

Introduction

Primary care trusts (PCTs) are new and evolving organizations. Although parts of their lineage can be traced to earlier forms of primary care-based organizations such as general practitioner (GP) fundholding, total purchasing and GP commissioning groups (Mays *et al.* 2001), their particular combination of size, governance and functions makes them very different from their predecessors. Even the change from primary care groups to PCTs has been described as a transformation rather than a transition (Robinson and Exworthy 2001). This newness and originality means that there are many aspects of PCTs that can be expected to change over time. In the light of this evolving agenda, this chapter looks at the international experience of primary care organizations to establish whether it holds any relevance for PCTs.

The chapter is organized into two main sections. The first section presents some of the salient features of primary care organizations in several countries that are often cited as comparators for the UK system. These are the social insurance-based (or Bismarck) systems found in France and Germany; the Nordic countries of Finland, Sweden, Norway and Denmark; New Zealand, where many reforms similar to those implemented in the UK were introduced in recent years; and the USA, where managed care plans have pioneered a range of micro-management techniques over the last two decades. The second section identifies several aspects of primary care organizations that have been developed in these countries and suggests that these may be helpful in considering the future development of PCTs.

It is important to emphasize at the outset, however, that this chapter is not an attempt to identify lessons for English PCTs from international experience. As I have argued elsewhere, the desire to draw lessons from abroad is a fashionable activity but a hazardous one (Robinson and Steiner 1998). The fact that countries embody very different histories, cultures and socio-economic institutions makes the export of ideas and evidence extremely problematic. These considerations apply with particular force in the case of primary care organization and performance. The aims of this chapter are, therefore, far more modest. In short, I aim to present available evidence about the approaches of some other countries, with a view to generating debate about the future development of primary care policy in England.

Primary care organizations around the world

Primary care in France and Germany

In comparison with England, primary care in France and Germany is characterized by four main features. There is a less clear distinction between primary care and outpatient or specialist ambulatory care; there are no fixed patient lists and no, or only limited, gatekeeping between primary and secondary care; there is a high degree of patient choice between providers; and payment of primary care practitioners is on a fee-for-service basis.

In France, ambulatory care is provided by both generalists and specialists practising privately. Most of these practitioners work alone. Patients have free choice of a doctor, regardless of specialty, and do not require a referral to see a specialist. However, this system has come under some criticism in recent years and, in 1997, a gatekeeping system based upon a referring doctor was introduced on a voluntary basis. General practitioners who adopt this system undertake to keep patient records, ensure continuity of care, engage in preventive health care programmes and comply with medical guidelines. To date, however, only about 10 per cent of GPs and 1 per cent of patients have accepted this system. As such, the system remains one of fragmented services, although considerable effort has been put into the development and dissemination of medical practice guidelines. Failure to comply with guidelines can result in financial penalties (Paris *et al.* 2002).

In Germany, office-based physicians also provide primary care. Slightly fewer than 40 per cent of them have been trained formally as GPs, while others are specialists in, for example, internal medicine, gynaecology and paediatrics. In addition to the approximately 113,000 office-based practitioners, there are about 11,000 physicians (often heads of hospital departments) who are authorized to treat ambulatory patients from their offices (Busse 2000). Because there is no gatekeeping function, patients are allowed to select a sickness fund-affiliated doctor of their choice – many patients consult office-based specialists rather than GPs. Despite efforts by the federal government to improve the status of family practice, over recent decades the number of office-based specialists has increased far more rapidly.

In terms of performance, the German system scores highly in relation to free choice of providers – this is highly regarded by patients and defended fiercely by physicians. However, within such a *laisser-faire* system, cost control is weak (particularly when costs are fuelled by fee-for-service payments) and coordination of care is difficult. Attempts have been made on the part of some sickness funds to improve coordination through selective contracting with designated primary and secondary care providers. These have focused on the provision of integrated care through chronic disease management programmes. However, progress has been slow. In general, payment systems and contracts provide few incentives for well coordinated care. Moreover, despite the fact that physicians' associations advise sickness funds on the allocation and prioritization of spending, there is no real primary care-based purchasing in Germany.

Primary care in the Nordic countries

The organization and finance of primary care in the Nordic countries is characterized by a high level of local government responsibility; thus there is strong local accountability. Considerable emphasis is also placed on the planned provision of services. The organization of care frequently manifests itself in a multidisciplinary approach – often embracing social services – and a strong gatekeeping function. General practitioners themselves are often private practitioners with strong contractual relations with local municipalities.

The Finnish health care system provides a good example of this approach. In this system, the main decision-making power rests with the 448 municipal councils that cover populations of, on average, 11,000 people (which range from less than 1,000 to over 500,000). Each council is elected every 4 years by local residents and appoints an executive board that is accountable to the council. The council also appoints members to various municipal committees, including health, education and social services. The municipal council, the municipal executive board and the committees are politically accountable to the electorate.

The health committee, in consultation with the municipal council and executive board, makes decisions on the planning and organization of health care. In recent years, two trends have become noticeable. First, there has been a tendency to devolve greater decision-making authority to key individuals within the committees. Secondly, a number of municipalities (38 per cent in 1999) had merged their social services and health committees in the interests of better coordination.

Within primary care, the main features of the current system of service organization were introduced in 1972. This is based upon a nationwide system of health centres. Municipalities run these and although their main function is to provide office-based general medical care, they tend to provide a wider range of curative, preventive and public health services. These will usually include outpatient medical care, some inpatient care (a typical health centre will have 30–60 beds, most of which are for elderly and chronically ill patients), maternity care, child health care, home nursing, school health care, care for the elderly, family planning, physiotherapy and rehabilitative care, occupational health care and dental care. The centres are usually well-equipped with consulting rooms for both doctors and nurses, X-ray facilities, clinical laboratories, facilities for minor surgery and endoscopy, and equipment such as electrocardiograms and ultrasound.

Health centres mainly serve populations of 10,000 patients and above (although some are smaller) and are designed to provide integrated, multidisciplinary care. A typical centre will employ GPs, some medical specialists, nurses, public health specialists, midwives, social workers, dentists and various therapists. The centres are managed either by a chief physician (in smaller centres) or by a management team comprising physicians, nurses and administrators in larger centres.

The centre acts as a gatekeeper to secondary care. Choice for patients between secondary care centres is not offered, although greater choice over health centre enrolments and hospitals is currently under discussion. However, in general, responsibility and planning for integrated services receive higher priority than consumer-led initiatives surrounding individual choice. At the same time, a marked feature of the Finnish system has been the emergence of local projects and experiments around the country. Several of these have been based on purchaser–provider models similar to those developed in the UK. For example, one municipality has decided to purchase its health services from Samfundet Folkhalsan, a not-for-profit private sector organization. In another municipality, that of Mantta, the primary care health centre and the hospital have merged into a single organization that provides all the health services for the local population and for the population of another nearby municipality as well. Because these arrangements are of recent origin, little evaluative evidence is available about their performance at the moment (Jarvelin 2002).

Primary care in Sweden and Norway is also organized at the local government level. In Sweden, county councils employ GPs in health centres on a salaried basis. Since 1995, all physicians in primary care have been required to specialize in general practice. They provide treatment and act as a guide for patients through the system. They do not, however, have a monopoly of primary care services. Patients may go directly to hospital outpatient departments or seek medical attention at private clinics that are usually publicly funded. Indeed, around half of all outpatient visits in Sweden are made to outpatient clinics rather than health centres, even though the user charge for such a visit (16–27 euros in 2000) is higher than the charge for a health centre consultation (6–13 euros). Another 25 per cent of consultations take place in privately run clinics that often have contracts with the county council (Hjortsberg and Ghatnekar 2001).

Another striking feature of the Swedish system is the special role of district nurses within health centres. They often carry out first-contact assessments in their own nursing rooms. They also have major responsibilities in home care and limited prescribing rights.

In Norway, the 435 municipalities have the responsibility for organizing primary care. In common with Sweden and Finland, the scope of primary care is wide and covers prevention, treatment, rehabilitation and nursing care. Around 80 per cent of GPs are private practitioners who contract with the municipality; the remainder are municipal employees. Given the importance attached to local government planning in the Norwegian health care system, it is somewhat surprising that a patient list system in primary care was not introduced until as late as 1997, and then only on a trial basis. However, since January 2001, primary care lists have been introduced nationwide and are expected to improve the organization and coordination of care (Furuholmen 2000).

In Denmark, municipal and county authorities also have responsibility for running health care services. However, more emphasis is currently being placed upon patient choice than in some of the other Nordic countries. As in the UK, GPs play an important role as gatekeepers to hospitals and specialist care. Some exceptions apply, such as direct access to ear, nose and throat specialists and to ophthalmologists, but in all other cases GP referrals are required. Since 1993, however, there has been a movement towards offering patients greater choice over hospital treatments. This has involved an entitlement to receive treatment at a hospital of choice anywhere in the country. General practitioners are an important source of advice for patients when making these decisions, although only about 2 per cent of patients have taken up this option to date. It is expected that over time, as choice becomes more established, stronger incentives will develop for hospitals to provide better information on waiting times and quality.

General practitioners are, in principle, private practitioners and about one-third of them are solo practitioners. However, the Ministry of Health is currently encouraging a move towards group practices to promote higher quality services through teamwork and better coordination. Better collaboration has resulted in 24-hour access to GP services in most parts of the country (Vallgarda *et al.* 2001).

Primary care in New Zealand

New Zealand is an interesting comparator because its course of recent health policy reform closely parallels that of the UK. Like the UK, it introduced a model based upon purchaser–provider separation and competition during the 1990s but, since 1999, has drawn back from this model. The incoming Labour/ Alliance government in 1999 held the view that the internal market had failed to deliver significant improvements in efficiency and quality, that it had imposed heavy transactions costs and that it had led to a loss of public confidence in the health care system. As a result, recent structural changes have blurred the purchaser–provider split and moved back to a more integrated approach. As in the UK, however, some of the primary care developments of the earlier period have been retained and are seen as holding potential for future service improvements.

The traditional model of primary care in New Zealand before 1993 was very similar to the traditional model in the UK. General practitioners were private practitioners, often operating as single-handed practices. They performed a gatekeeping function and referred patients to secondary care providers. Unlike the UK, patients were charged a fee for consultations and so the business ethic was possibly stronger than in the UK. In 1993, however, what has been described as a cultural revolution began. In response to the Health and Disabilities Services Act, GPs started to organize themselves into independent practitioner associations. These were usually within defined geographical areas and ranged in size from six to eight GPs to groupings of up to 340 GPs. Some of the independent practitioner associations were allocated budgets for managing pharmaceuticals and diagnostic testing. This represented a more limited form of UK-style GP fundholding. Any savings could be used to fund local health initiatives. Savings realized in this way have been used to introduce information management and quality assurance systems, to run continuing education courses for their members and to launch various initiatives around integrated care.

The growth of the independent practitioner associations has superimposed a more corporate structure on general practice in New Zealand. It has provided scope for collaborative working among previously fragmented and atomistic general practices. In 1999, over 80 per cent of GPs were members of independent practitioner associations. Some independent practitioner associations have been particularly active in the development of integrated care programmes. These may involve merged funding schemes, devolved purchasing responsibilities, close cooperation between different agencies and the provision of coordinated care for defined populations. The central health funding authority has funded ten demonstration projects designed to provide integrated care to specified populations. These extend from a scheme in Canterbury to integrate services for older people across primary, secondary and community care to an integrated care initiative for diabetes management. The development and use of common clinical guidelines is an important feature of these schemes.

Building on these experiences, a primary care strategy published in 2001 announced the creation of primary health organizations. These comprise teams of primary care providers and emphasize a team approach, with a strong emphasis on preventive care. They are not-for-profit bodies that manage per capita funding for enrolled patients. The first primary health organization was established in July 2002 covering deprived populations of Maori and Pacific Islanders. Primary health organizations offer an organizational structure, with many similarities to English PCTs, for developing integrated care schemes on an even wider basis (French *et al.* 2001).

Primary care in the USA

The USA does not have a strong tradition of primary care. The 'first contact' aspect of primary care is often seen as a threat to free choice and incompatible with a competitive, market approach to the delivery of health services (Starfield 1994). Nonetheless, concern with ever-rising health care costs, often driven by supplier-induced demand, led to the dramatic expansion during the 1980s and 1990s of various kinds of managed care organizations. These take many forms, but are essentially insurance organizations that act as purchasing agents on behalf of those individuals enrolled with them. Unlike the traditional US fee-for-service system, managed care organizations have populations defined by enrolment in the plan; restricted patient choice over secondary care providers; fixed payment schemes for providers (such as hospitals and doctors) that are independent of use; and methods for controlling health service utilization and doctors' practices (Robinson and Steiner 1998). Managed care organizations, therefore, perform many of the functions performed by primary care organizations in other countries.

During the 1990s, managed care approaches were vigorously marketed around the world as a method of coordinating care and containing costs (Rosleff and Lister 1995; Woods 1997). Somewhat ironically, this export effort was taking place when disenchantment was spreading in the USA about the performance of managed care. Allegations of falling quality standards, restricted access to services and rising insurance premiums were the major causes of concern (Saltman 1998; Robinson 2000). One analyst (Robinson 2001) has proclaimed the end of managed care in the USA, a consequence of economic success but political failure (meaning that cost reductions and efficiency gains were achieved, but the consequences of restricted access resulted in a backlash from the public and politicians that led to the curtailment of managed care). Notwithstanding these concerns, and whatever the future of managed care in the USA, it is still possible to point to several aspects of the managed care approach that have attracted attention beyond the USA and been applied with some success in other health care systems.

In particular, managed care organizations have developed several micro-management techniques for managing clinical behaviour. The main techniques are utilization review and management, provider profiling and disease management. Utilization review and management form the crux of the managed care approach. In essence, utilization review seeks to reduce unnecessary or inappropriate care by scrutinizing past, current and planned use of services. Its main forms are prospective utilization review or pre-authorization through which a clinician or patient must receive approval for a service before it is provided; concurrent review, which assesses the progress of care against defined plans in relation to, for example, hospital lengths of stay and ancillary service use; and retrospective review, which involves auditing patient records and claims. Utilization review is an aggressive technique, challenging to both clinicians and the *status quo*. This is, no doubt, part of the reason why it is alleged by some clinicians to be inefficient and ineffective. It is, however, undoubtedly the most widely used managed care technique, so much so that many fee-for-service plans now also employ utilization review.

Provider profiling involves the statistical analysis of performance in terms of defined criteria. It may be applied at the individual or organizational level and has much in common with the standard industrial practice of benchmarking (Grout *et al.* 2000). In the case of individual physician profiling, attention may, for example, focus on patients' length of stay in hospital. Data on the performance of all physicians within a specialty will be collected and an individual physician's performance will be compared with the norm. On the basis of this information, attempts may be made to modify the clinical behaviour of certain physicians whose practice differs from the norm for no transparent reason. To work effectively, profiling requires considerable investments in information systems that permit, *inter alia*, reliable case-mix adjustments. In fact, the USA has made considerable strides in the development of information technology systems, including those covering the quality of care (Enthoven 1999).

Disease management entails the development of integrated packages of care across the whole spectrum of a particular disease. The approach is applied particularly in the case of chronic illnesses such as diabetes, asthma and heart disease, where risk identification, diagnosis, preventive care, treatment and on-going monitoring take place over an extended period of time. Within the disease management approach, an important feature is the production of care plans and having providers work to these through the use of guidelines and protocols.

One of the largest and most well-known managed care organizations in the USA is the Kaiser Permanente plan with 6.1 million members in California and another 2.1 million members in other states. Feacham *et al.* (2002) have studied the relative performance of the Kaiser plan in relation to the UK's National Health Service (NHS). Their conclusion that Kaiser obtained better performance than the NHS at roughly the same cost has attracted widespread criticism. Nonetheless, they do point to several aspects of the Kaiser managed care approach, involving many of the techniques outlined above, that have relevance for the UK.

First, Kaiser achieves a high degree of integration across all components of the healthcare system. This enables patients to be managed in the most appropriate settings, disease management programmes for chronic conditions to be implemented, and expenditure trade-offs to be made in terms of appropriateness and cost-effectiveness rather than being constrained by artificial budget categories. Secondly, as a direct result of its integrated approach, Kaiser is able to control hospital admission rates and lengths of stay. As a result, Kaiser members spend about one-third of the time in hospital currently spent by NHS patients. Thirdly, Kaiser has a sophisticated and efficient information technology system that reduces time spent on administrative tasks, especially time spent by clinicians taking medical histories, dictating letters and locating patient records. Kaiser spends about 2 per cent of its total budget on information technology, whereas the NHS plans to spend about 0.5 per cent of its budget on information technology over the next few years (see Chapter 8).

International experience and primary care trusts

The preceding section has outlined some of the main features of the organization, finance and delivery of primary care in a selection of countries often cited as comparators for the UK as far as health policy is concerned. What is the relevance of this international experience for English PCTs?

The first point to make is that, unlike some areas of health care where the UK is often described to be lagging behind other countries, in primary care the UK is almost certainly a world leader. The well-developed system of general practice with its close-to-universal coverage, the continuity achieved through its lists of registered patients and its system of referrals to secondary care is widely seen as a model to which many other countries aspire.

Moreover, primary care-based purchasing has progressed far further in the UK than in almost any other country, certainly much further than in any other European country. Admittedly, a form of GP fundholding has been developed in the Catalonia region of Spain; in 2001 there were seven primary care teams of doctors and nurses receiving budgets covering diagnostic tests, specialist referrals and pharmaceuticals for defined populations of 50,000 to 100,000 people. Since 1998, family practitioners in Estonia have also been delegated limited fundholding responsibilities. There have also been fundholding experiments in Imola (near Bologna in Italy) and in St Petersburg in the Russian Federation during the 1990s. Nevertheless, none of these countries has a nationwide system of primary care organizations that have been delegated budgetary responsibility for the purchase of secondary care services on the scale that PCTs have been allocated budgets in England (McCallum *et al.*, in press).

Finally, the organizational structure represented by PCTs is far more advanced in its attempt to manage and coordinate primary care delivery within a corporate framework than has been achieved in most other countries. The emerging corporate nature of PCTs offers more scope for improving clinical standards through clinical governance than exists in other, more dispersed systems. Moreover, the fragmentation of primary care services remains a major problem in many countries. Taken together, the nature of primary care provision in England, its purchasing role and its emerging corporate structure, probably means that other countries may have more to learn from PCTs than England has to learn from them!

However, it would be wrong to be too complacent. Although the PCT experiment may be at the forefront of organizational development in primary care, there are nonetheless a number of areas highlighted by international experience that are worth noting in relation to future primary care policy development. These include the role of patient choice, local accountability, micro-management techniques and service integration, and the use of pilot schemes and experimentation.

Patient choice

The introduction of greater patient choice figures prominently in the English government's future aspirations for the NHS. The limited choice offered in numerous areas of the health service contrasts vividly with the growth of consumer choice in many other areas of everyday life. In France and Germany, as the preceding section of this chapter explained, choice of doctors – including direct access to specialists – is a highly valued feature of these systems. In the Netherlands, patients have choice over the sickness funds with which they register and which purchase care on their behalf. In the USA, choice between both insurance plans and providers has always been a highly valued aspect of the system. Managed care sought to restrict this choice and this is cited as one reason for its demise, as consumerism reasserts itself (Robinson 2001).

Primary care trusts as currently structured do not offer patients choice over the organization that will organize care and purchase it on their behalf. Primary care trusts have geographically defined catchment areas and patients who live in these areas are automatically assigned to the relevant trust. There is some scope for offering choice of a secondary care provider, in consultation with the referring GP, but quite how far this will be developed is difficult to anticipate. The government's response to this dilemma seems to be to offer greater choice at the margins (walk-in clinics, NHS Direct, rights to choose public or private providers in the event of cancelled operations) rather than to address the fundamental structural limitations created by the geographical monopoly exercised by PCTs.

Of course, not everyone will be bothered by the lack of choice offered by PCTs. As in the Nordic countries, some limitation on choice is the price that is paid for population-based approaches to health care and coordinated service provision. In these systems, patient 'voice' (influence through the political/administrative process) is substituted for patient 'exit' (the classic market mechanism of choosing not to buy) as a driver of patient-responsive services. However, despite the considerable effort put into the establishment of PCT boards, with lay members who are meant to be representative of their local communities, there is still something of a democratic deficit compared with the Nordic experience (see also Chapter 11).

Local accountability

Finland provides an example of a country with strong local accountability through the political system. As pointed out above, locally elected councils appoint members to municipal committees that are responsible for health and other local services. At the same time, however, the needs of modern management are being recognized, through greater devolution of decision-making authority to local health centre management teams.

Primary care trusts face a similar need to balance managerial and political imperatives. The presence of executive and non-executive or lay members on their boards, with the latter often having local political affiliations, is one aspect of the quest for balance. The decision to appoint a professional executive committee, in addition to a board, suggests recognition of the need to enlist GP support within a network-based organization. Whether this structure will succeed in delivering the required local accountability, particularly when its responsibility for the allocation of a major part of the secondary care purchasing budget becomes transparent, remains to be seen.

Micro-management techniques and service integration

Primary care trusts face a huge challenge in reducing inappropriate variations in clinical practice and in improving service standards, particularly through better integration between primary, secondary and social care. It is so often a breakdown at the interfaces between these service areas that leads to poor patient care. The NHS has made enormous strides in improving performance in this regard through numerous national initiatives, including national service frameworks and performance management methods. Substantial progress has been made through the development of integrated care programmes in areas such as diabetes and asthma care, and through the introduction of clinical governance more generally (see Chapter 7).

The review of international evidence presented here suggests that an agent or agency acting on the patient's behalf is likely to be important in developing integrated care packages. Primary care professionals acting as gatekeepers are obviously well placed to perform this role. In this connection, Boerma *et al.* (1997) assessed the services offered by GPs in 30 European countries. Their results confirm that in those countries with a strong gatekeeping function, such as Denmark, the Netherlands and the UK, GPs have a significantly enhanced position as the doctor of first contact. Clearly, this places them in a strong position also to act as the patient's agent in the coordination of care packages. But gatekeeping may be a necessary but not sufficient condition for better coordination. Certainly, Boerma *et al.* (1997) found no significant correlation between gatekeeping and disease management (defined as the management and follow-up of a broad range of acute and chronic diseases) or preventive medicine (including hypertensive, cholesterol and cervical cancer screening, child immunization and health education).

It may be that the agency relationship needs to be defined more broadly than GP-based gatekeeping. The preceding review has discussed the role of managed care in the USA. It has been argued that, despite the general disenchantment with this approach in the USA, managed care has nonetheless pioneered many micro-management techniques that can be applied with success in non-US contexts. In fact, various forms of utilization management, profiling and disease management have already been applied with considerable success by English primary care organizations (Robinson and Steiner 1998; Mays *et al.* 2001). But there is scope for far more development in this direction. Reference has already been made to the achievements of Kaiser Permanente in the USA, with its emphasis on good information systems and an integrated care approach. An added salience has been given to this experience by discussions that have taken place at ministerial level about US and other overseas providers being given the opportunity to manage English PCTs on a contractual basis.

Pilot schemes and experimentation

Primary care has gone through a revolution in the UK over the last 10 years. Wave upon wave of organizational changes have been introduced. Often these have been introduced nationwide over very short time-scales. The introduction of PCTs is a classic example of this trend. Untried organizations have been set up, with policy and operating procedures developed on the hoof. In these circumstances, it is not so much a surprise that many organizations struggle with, for example, inadequate management capacity (such as the severe shortage of senior finance management skills – see Chapter 6), but that they have managed to cope as well as they have.

This way of doing things is far more unusual in other countries. There appears to be a far greater willingness to pilot new schemes and evaluate performance before undertaking wholesale change. Examples have been provided of local demonstration projects in both Finland and New Zealand. In the USA, too, demonstration projects and evaluation are a standard feature of federally funded schemes, although in addition the wide diversity within the US system means that there are many natural experiments available for evaluative research. Just as the trend in the UK is towards evidence-based clinical practice, there is clearly a case for more attention to evidence – before wide-scale change – in the primary care policy area.

Conclusions

This chapter did not aim to derive lessons for the UK from international experience. This is just as well, because the UK has probably less to learn from other countries in relation to primary care than it does in relation to many other areas of health care. The well-established GP system, with its universal coverage, patient lists and gatekeeping function provides a far stronger foundation for comprehensive coordination of care than exists in most other countries.

Beyond this, the particular form of corporate, networked organization represented by PCTs is a more complex and ambitious form of primary care organization than exists in most other countries. It presents challenges in terms of intra-organization leadership and management, as well as inter-organizational coordination, which are very different to those found elsewhere. At the same time, however, as the review in this chapter shows, international experience does highlight issues surrounding patient choice, local accountability, service integration and local experimentation that will need to be addressed in the course of the future development of PCTs.

References

Boerma, W., van der Zee, J. and Fleming, D. (1997) Service profiles of general practitioners in Europe, *British Journal of General Practice*, 47: 481–6.

Busse, R. (2000) *Health Care Systems in Transition: Germany*. Copenhagen: European Observatory on Health Care Systems.

Enthoven, A. (1999) *In Pursuit of an Improving National Health Service*. London: Nuffield Trust.

Feacham, R., Sekhri, N. and White, K. (2002) Getting more for their dollar: a comparison of the NHS with California's Kaiser Permanente, *British Medical Journal*, 324(733): 135–43.

French, S., Old, A. and Healy, J. (2001) *Health Care Systems in Transition: New Zealand*. Copenhagen: European Observatory on Health Care Systems.

Furuholmen, C. (2000) *Health Care Systems in Transition: Norway*. Copenhagen: European Observatory on Health Care Systems.

Grout, P., Jenkins, A. and Propper, C. (2000) *Benchmarking and Incentives in the NHS*. London: Office of Health Economics.

Hjortsberg, C. and Ghatnekar, O. (2001) *Health Care Systems in Transition: Sweden*. Copenhagen: European Observatory on Health Care Systems.

Jarvelin, J. (2002) *Healthcare Systems in Transition: Finland*. Copenhagen: European Observatory on Health Care Systems.

Mays, N., Wyke, S., Malbon, G. and Goodwin, N. (eds) (2001) *The Purchasing of Health Care by Primary Care Organizations: An Evaluation and Guide to Future Policy*. Buckingham: Open University Press.

McCallum, A., Brommels, M., Robinson, R., Bergman, S. and Palu, T. (in press) The impact of primary care purchasing in Europe, in R. Saltman and A. Rico (eds) *Primary Care in the Driver's Seat: Organizational Reform in European Primary Care*. Buckingham: Open University Press.

Paris, V., Polton, D. and Sandier, S. (2002) *Health Care Systems in Transition: France*. Copenhagen: European Observatory on Health Care Systems.

Robinson, J. (2001) The end of managed care, *Journal of the American Medical Association*, 285(20): 2622–8.

Robinson, R. (2000) Managed health care: a dilemma for evidence-based policy; *Health Economics*, 9(1): 1–7.

Robinson, R. and Exworthy, M. (2001) *Three at the Top*. Report prepared for the NHS Leadership Centre. London: London School of Economics and Political Science.

Robinson, R. and Steiner, A. (1998) *Managed Health Care*. Buckingham: Open University Press.

Rosleff, F. and Lister, G. (1995) *European Healthcare Trends: Towards Managed Care in Europe*. London: Coopers & Lybrand.

Saltman, R. (1998) The sad saga of managed care in the United States, *Eurohealth*, 4(2): 35–6.

Starfield, B. (1994) Is primary care essential, *Lancet*, 344(8930): 1129–33.

Vallgarda, S., Krasnik, A. and Vrangbaek, K. (2001) *Health Care Systems in Transition: Denmark*. Copenhagen: European Observatory on Health Care Systems.

Woods, D. (1997) *The Future of the Managed Care Industry*. London: Economist Intelligence Unit.

4 Primary care organizations, inequalities and equity

Deborah Baker

Introduction

One of the founding objectives of primary care trusts (PCTs) is to improve the health of, and address inequalities in, their communities (Secretary of State for Health 1997). This involves making decisions about what are the most important inequalities in a particular locality and delivering improvements in the quality and efficiency of care for local populations. The assumption is that health professionals working locally will be most knowledgeable about the priorities that should be set and thus best placed to recommend the appropriate actions needed to improve health and reduce inequality for their particular populations. These are noble sentiments, but they raise several questions; these may appear at first sight to be academic, but nevertheless have crucial implications for how local policies are prioritized and implemented.

In this chapter, I argue that the focus on improving population health and reducing inequality disguises two linked but fundamentally different agendas – attaining equity in the distribution of health care and attaining equality in the distribution of health. Initially, I consider the concept of equity and its implications for the distribution of health care in relation to need. I then move on to discuss what relevance primary care has for tackling health inequality and the dilemmas that face PCT policy-makers in deciding which health inequalities matter most in their localities and the best means of resolving them. The focus in this section will be on preventive medicine. Finally, I briefly evaluate the state of the inequalities agenda in PCTs to date.

Inequity in the distribution of health care

The concepts of inequity and inequality are by no means synonymous; while inequality is in its simplest sense a measurement of variation between populations or individuals, inequity carries a normative or value-laden connotation as to whether identified inequalities are unjust (Gwatkin 2000). Concern for the just distribution of health care is epitomized in a principle that has wide acceptance in the National Health Service (NHS) – the goal of equitable distribution of health care in relation to population need. However, for this to be translated into action in specific localities, it is important to consider how 'need' is defined and measured; which aspects of service provision are currently most inequitably distributed; and the policies that have, in the past, led to a more equitable distribution of resources.

The meaning of 'population need'

Perhaps the most rational basis for deciding what constitutes 'population need' is that proposed by Sen (1982), whereby need is defined in relation to the health care required to maintain normal functioning; each according to their need for functioning. Need in this sense is conceptualized as the ability to flourish or to attain one's potential as a human being. Disease or dysfunction restricts access to life's opportunities to which all of us have an equal right, but health care can keep us functioning as close to the norm as possible (Daniels *et al.* 1996; Olsen 1997). Implicit in this definition, as Culyer (2001) has pointed out, is that the need for health services is contingent on the knowledge that these services will actually improve health, prevent its deterioration or postpone death – in other words, that they are effective.

Although this definition of need makes rational sense, it presents a number of dilemmas for PCTs if they are to distribute resources equitably in relation to population need. The most obvious of these difficulties is that PCTs are limited in their ability to meet the need for health care by scarcity of resources and levels of technological development. In this context, 'fairness' implies the distribution of health care proportional to people's needs, so that those with like needs should receive like attention and resources (i.e. horizontal equity) and those with greater needs should receive greater attention and resources (i.e. vertical equity) (Mooney 1983; Culyer 2001). How to decide what constitutes 'greater need' thus becomes central to the concern for the equitable allocation of resources. Most usually, 'greater need' is directly equated with relative deprivation, given the overwhelming evidence of poorer health for those with lower socio-economic status. But, as Marchand *et al.* (1998) suggest, those who are threatened with the worst harms, who have the shortest life expectancy and experience the most serious diseases and injuries should count as the 'worst off'. This is a more inclusive focus, as it can also embrace other social and demographic sources of need such as age, gender and ethnicity.

Assessment of the need for primary care

Needs assessment has historically been a basic component in providing appropriate secondary care provision in England. Conventionally, population need is assessed using composite indices that combine several socio-economic and/or demographic proxy indictors in a single score. However, the methods used in the construction of such indices render them problematic for locality-based needs assessment that can inform levels of primary care provision. The most fundamental problem is that of determining which combination of indicators best reflects different dimensions of need and then devising an appropriate method for assigning weights so that indicators can be combined. The durability of such weights, particularly over time and in relation to local contexts, is questionable (Carr-Hill *et al.* 1998).

This is well illustrated by use of the Jarman Index as a means of identifying localities with the greatest need for primary care (Jarman 1983). The Jarman Index (Jarman 1991) is the only needs-based formula that is currently applied in primary care settings. It is used to determine the level of additional remuneration for general practices that operate in areas where workload is increased due to high levels of need. Wisely, Jarman compiled the index using eight indicators, reflecting different sources of need in the community (elderly people living alone, children under five, ethnic minority groups, single-parent households, membership of lowest social class V, unemployment, people living in overcrowded housing, and people changing address within 1 year), rather than focusing exclusively on the need associated with material deprivation. Nevertheless, the particular combination of Jarman's indicators and the weightings assigned to them has meant an overestimation of need associated with deprivation (Carr-Hill and Sheldon 1991; Senior 1991) and the neglect of other sources of need, such as age and ethnicity.

Hann and Baker (2002) have demonstrated this effect using primary care group/trust (PCG/T) populations. Separate indices for age/sex, deprivation and ethnicity were used to 'profile' need, and the relationship between levels of need ascertained by these indices and those predicted by the Jarman Index was examined. The analysis revealed that the Jarman Index identified high levels of need associated with deprivation, but not areas with high age-related need or less deprived areas with ethnically mixed populations (Senior 1991; Baker *et al.* 1994). The problems with composite needs indices suggest that local needs profiling by PCTs based on easily available and regularly updatable information would be preferable to opaque and statistically complex derived indices (Carr-Hill and Sheldon 1992; Sheldon *et al.* 1993).

A similar concern has recently been voiced in the initial planning stages of a 'health/poverty index', in which a wide variety of NHS, academic, local authority and voluntary organizations were consulted to identify and assess options and methods for developing the index (Dibben *et al.* 2001). Participants acknowledged that single composite indices had utility at the macro (national, regional or health authority) level, acting as general indicators of health, poverty and deprivation. However, indices that could not be broken down into their component parts for smaller areas were not helpful for the purposes of needs assessment.

Another challenge facing PCTs is that health and sickness are culturally contingent, so that the circumstances and attributes needed to 'flourish' in Britain today may vary between different social groups. This involves not just a consideration about overall levels of resources, but also whether the nature of the resources available is appropriate to meet the needs of particular social groups.

Access to primary care

Access is an issue that is at the heart of equity in the distribution of health care. Any impediments that discriminate between patients or that prevent access will create inequity. At its most basic, access reflects availability; if services are not available, then they cannot be used. A failure of primary care equitably to match the needs of local populations has been consistently manifested in poorer access for more needy groups – the 'inverse care law' (Tudor Hart 1971). But it is a mistake to regard the 'inverse care law' as universally applicable to all aspects of primary care or, even where it does apply, to assume that it remains inviolate over time.

There is some evidence to suggest that an incentive payment for the provision of specific services reduces inequity in their distribution. Incentives introduced in the 1990 general practitioner (GP) contract have meant that fee-for-service, supply-led services, such as minor surgery, child health surveillance and chronic disease management for asthma and diabetes, are now widely available, so that inverse care is visible only in some parts of the country, in particular London (Baker and Hann 2001). Inequities in the coverage of cervical screening and immunization between affluent and deprived areas have also narrowed since an incentive payment for meeting targets was introduced (Middleton and Baker 2003; Baker and Middleton 2003). Equity in the use of primary care services (GP consultation) relative to need also appears close to becoming a reality, as barriers to accessing primary care physicians have largely been overcome (van Doorslaer *et al.* 2000; Baker *et al.* 2002).

Some variations in access, however, remain. The unequal distribution of primary care physicians and other health professionals in relation to population need has persisted over the last decade (Benzeval and Judge 1996; Gravelle and Sutton 2001). There are also wide variations in access to appropriate and high-quality care that are determined by the clinical judgements and preferences of physicians and by the organization of care at the GP surgery (McPherson *et al.* 1982; Leese and Bosanquet 1995; Lynch 1995). In these instances, it is still important to determine whether variation is in fact inequit-able, in the sense that it severely restricts access to services that will affect 'the capacity to maintain normal functioning' for those in most need.

This qualification risks being overlooked in the general current emphasis on quality improvement. For example, there are currently overarching con-cerns about waiting times before receiving an appointment with a GP and it is a national priority to ensure that patients do not have to wait more than 48 hours to see their doctor. However, there is little evidence of the inequity of GP utilization in relation to need that severely affects functioning (Baker *et al.* 2002). On the other hand, there is a preponderance of female GPs in affluent rather than deprived areas and this restricts the choice of women in more disadvantaged areas to see a GP of their own sex (Hann and Baker 2002). The presence of a female GP has been associated with higher uptake of screening in general practice (Majeed *et al.* 1994; Ibbotson *et al.* 1996), but the distribution of female GPs does not generally feature as a central part of PCT initiatives to address either inequality or quality of care.

Inequality in the distribution of health

Equity, with its connotations of social justice, is a concept that becomes much more problematic if it is used to make judgements about which inequalities in health matter most and should, therefore, be a priority for action at the local level. The question as to whether inequalities in health are in fact inequitable is difficult to resolve, because what is 'fair' or 'just' in this context is not always obvious. One widely held view is that inequalities become inequitable when people have little control over the causes of inequality – the social determin-ants of disease and death. Le Grand (1982) argues that the element that is crucial to determining the fairness or otherwise of health inequalities is the existence of choice. According to this argument, health inequalities are based on structural and material factors that are beyond the control of the indi-vidual. For example, the incomes people receive are strongly influenced (if not completely determined) by factors about which individuals have no choices. Thus health inequalities that are associated with income inequalities are necessarily unjust.

Such an approach, however, takes no account of the factors that mediate the relation between income and health in contemporary western societies – lifestyles associated with smoking and a diet rich in saturated fats and low in fresh fruit and vegetables. These behaviours and their consequences for health are not always part and parcel of being poor. In some European countries, for instance France and Spain, there is no association between socio-economic status and ischaemic heart disease and in others (for example, Portugal) the rates are actually lower for poorer people (Kunst *et al.* 1998). In England, there was no association between smoking and social class in the 1950s, despite considerable income inequality (Townsend 1995). Inequality in smoking behaviour only developed during the latter half of the twentieth century as a consequence of more rapid smoking cessation in affluent groups in response to health education messages. The adoption of such behaviours is not likely to be solely explained by income; rates of smoking cessation suggest that people do exert control over behaviours associated with poorer health.

The knotty moral question as to whether those engaging in unhealthy lifestyles should be held responsible for their poorer health should not enter into considerations of appropriate policies to reduce health inequality in the primary care context, since this issue could equally well be used to justify differential treatment as to identify inequities. If there are to be locality-based strategies to tackle inequality, these should, in the first instance, be firmly based on avoidance and targetted at those health inequalities that are avoidable, given appropriate primary care.

Reducing health inequality via primary care

The question as to whether health care can reduce health inequality would, within the conventional paradigms of research on health inequalities, be answered with a resounding 'no'. This is because of the belief that the fundamental causes of health inequality have their foundations in inequality in wealth, which directly or indirectly determines inequality in health outcomes. If this is the case, then even if it were possible to reduce inequality in access to and use of health services, this would have little effect on health outcomes without a concomitant redistribution of wealth. McKeown's (1979) treatise is a cornerstone of this argument. McKeown showed that improvements in standards of living and nutrition were responsible for the substantial decline in mortality from infectious diseases in Victorian and Edwardian England. This trend pre-dated the introduction of antibiotics; moreover, public health measures played only a marginal role. However, this evidence has now been subject to rigorous scrutiny and is less convincing as a consequence.

Szreter (1988) re-analysed McKeown's (1979) data, taking into account new evidence on long-term movements in average life expectancy, stretching back to pre-industrial Britain, and on urban/rural differences in mortality. Szreter (1988) demonstrated a primary role for public health measures in combatting the early nineteenth-century upsurge of diseases directly resulting from defective and unsanitary urban environments created in the course of industrialization. In this period, public health was part of local government rather than the health service, and social and medical interventions were unevenly implemented and only weakly centralized. Nevertheless, Szreter (1988) concluded that these were the principal source of improvement in the nation's health before the First World War, demonstrating that interventionist social welfare and health policies are creditable methods for improving the health of those living in poverty.

Mackenbach (1996) examined trends in mortality decline in the Netherlands in the nineteenth century, before and after the introduction of antibiotics. It was shown that the decline in mortality from infectious diseases more than doubled in pace after the introduction of antibiotics, thus highlighting the role of health care in accelerating the rate of health improvement. Mackenbach (1996), like Szreter (1988), also pointed to the role of public health in declining mortality; in the Netherlands, the public health movement promoted improvements in personal hygiene, birth control and sanitary living conditions through means as diverse as the educational system, societies founded 'to promote the public good' and welfare clinics for infants.

This evidence suggests a dual role for primary care in addressing health inequality: one is preventive action aimed at social causes that are directly modifiable by health care interventions; the other is preventive interventions to improve outcomes for disadvantaged groups, without necessarily being able to address the social determinants of poorer health.

Avoidable disease and death

The concept of avoidable mortality, in which conditions are identified that are amenable to medical or surgical treatment (Rutstein *et al.* 1976; Charlton and Velez 1986) is a good starting point for considering action that can be taken to tackle health inequalities in the primary care setting. Tobias and Jackson (2001) have recently extended this concept to include not only those causes of death amenable to therapeutic intervention, but also those responsive to individual and population-based preventive interventions. Based on this premise, Tobias and Jackson distinguished three main levels of intervention. Primary prevention describes action taken to prevent a condition developing by addressing its risk or protective factors, whether through individual behaviour change (such as lifestyle modification) or population intervention (such as public health policy). Secondary prevention focuses on conditions that respond to early detection and intervention, typically in a primary health care setting. As well as clinical preventive services such as cancer screening, secondary prevention includes chronic disease management intended to delay the progression of diseases such as diabetes or the recurrence of events such as heart attacks or stroke (for example, through the monitoring and management of high blood pressure). Finally, tertiary prevention includes those conditions whose case fatality rate can be reduced significantly by existing medical or surgical treatments (typically, but not necessarily in a hospital setting), even when the disease process is fully developed.

Tobias and Jackson (2001) then examined patterns of avoidable mortality in New Zealand from 1981 to 1987 and considered which level of preventive services would be most likely to reduce health inequalities. They demonstrated that the level varied according to whether inequalities were associated with gender, ethnicity or socio-economic status. For example, variations in avoidable mortality by gender were largely attributable to a higher incidence of conditions that are amenable to primary prevention in males. The largest variations in health by ethnicity were for conditions that were amenable to secondary prevention. These included conditions such as diabetes and cancers that are detected by screening (where the rates are over twice as common in both Maori and Pacific people than whites). All are amenable to early intervention and ongoing management in primary care settings. Socio-economic gradients in cause-specific mortality spanned the majority of avoidable mortalities and are therefore open to all three types of prevention. Tobias and Jackson concluded that:

> Both chronic disease and injury (and their respective risk and protective factors) must therefore be targeted by policies designed to reduce the toll of avoidable deaths. While medical treatment could achieve considerable health gain, primary preventive services (such as reducing smoking and improving diet and physical activity) and secondary preventive services (such as management of high blood pressure, diabetes and cancer screening) appear to hold the key to substantive reductions in these causes of death.
>
> (Tobias and Jackson 2001: 18)

Health inequality and preventive medicine

Despite Tobias and Jackson's (2001) analysis, little research has evaluated the effectiveness of primary care in achieving reductions in health inequality at the population level by means of the primary and secondary preventive services described above. Indeed, it is often assumed that such interventions increase inequality because affluent groups adopt healthier lifestyles faster than the less well off (Hart 1986; Reading *et al.* 1994). However, it is vitally important to view the impact of preventive interventions as a historical process, rather than through measurable 'before' and 'after' effects. Based on studies of child health in Brazil, Victora *et al.* (2000) proposed the 'inverse equity' hypothesis to demonstrate how inequality can change after the introduction of a preventive intervention. A new intervention is first picked up by the wealthy and, as a consequence, the outcome improves rapidly among this group because high coverage is reached within a short time. The outcome measure then stabilizes at a very low level among the wealthy, since no further reductions are possible – the minimum achievable plateau has been reached. The outcome then improves among the poor, but more slowly than it did among the wealthy, since uptake of the intervention is slower and there is greater scope for improvement due to the higher baseline level; at this stage the inequity gap narrows. Victora *et al*. (2000) emphasize that a fundamental issue in evaluating the impact of preventive interventions on inequality is the timing, since apparently contradictory results may be found at different stages of implementation.

This model was used to examine inequality in the coverage of preventive interventions and the implications for health outcomes among affluent and deprived health authorities in the UK in the 1990s. Two contrasting preventive measures, cervical screening and immunization for measles, mumps and rubella, were compared (Middleton and Baker 2003; Baker and Middleton, 2003). Over the decade, coverage was consistently higher in affluent areas for both interventions, but there was a decrease in inequality between affluent and deprived areas that echoed the final stage in the inverse equity hypothesis proposed by Victora *et al*. (2000).

Improved coverage in deprived areas was directly associated with changes in the organization of primary care, such as an increase in the number of practice nurses, fewer practising GPs over retirement age and better organization of call–recall systems at the practice level. Reductions in inequality in the coverage of cervical cytology screening in England had an impact on health inequality, particularly for women aged 35–64 years. There were strong correlations between higher achievement of cervical screening targets and lower incidence of cervical cancer in the deprived areas; from 1991 to 1997, incidence rates fell by 21 per cent for this age group in deprived health authorities, compared with 16 per cent in affluent health authorities. On the other hand, there were no significant differences in notifications for measles, mumps and rubella between affluent and deprived areas; notifications are now so low for these diseases in England that the link between their occurrence and changing patterns of immunization was not discernible at the macro level.

The implications for primary care trusts

From one perspective, this research is encouraging, since it illustrates that preventive interventions based in primary care can reduce health inequality. But from another perspective, it simply flags up the conflicting priorities faced by PCTs if they are actively to pursue the goal of reducing health inequalities in their localities.

First, the kind of interventions considered were those aimed at improving health for the whole of the eligible population. The resulting decrease in health inequality thus occurred almost as a side-effect of this activity (Petticrew and MacIntyre 2001), illustrating a 'top-down' strategy whereby reductions in ill-health in more affluent groups are followed only later by improvements in conditions among the poor (Gwatkin 2000). However, a concern for the efficiency of health systems – bringing about improvements in health conditions for the population as a whole – can conflict with policies whose aim is to focus on health improvement for the most disadvantaged groups. This is often referred to as the 'efficiency/equity trade-off' (Williams 2001). It implies that if PCTs wish to create more equality in health within their localities, some sacrifices may need to be made in terms of aggregate health gain. As can be seen in the examples given above, the general goal of efficiency means a delay in health improvement in areas with more deprived populations, although cervical screening and immunization did eventually improve population health and reduce inequality.

It would not be wise to draw general conclusions from this evidence, since the examples of preventive medicine described above have a direct impact on outcomes and this has implications for their effectiveness in tackling health inequality. Cervical cancer can be prevented by identification and treatment of abnormal cells by the Pap smear; infectious diseases can be curtailed though immunization. The accessibility of screening is potentially a source of inequality, but the intervention is not otherwise reliant for its success on eliminating the social determinants of these conditions. The issue that PCTs would need to address in relation to such interventions is how to redress the balance of inequality at an earlier time, so that the most disadvantaged groups are not the last to benefit from an intervention. This involves policies that focus on improving health outcomes faster and earlier for the most disadvantaged groups – a 'bottom-up' strategy. It also involves identifying those groups that are least likely to take up screening – a process that may well be specific to particular localities – and establishing those factors that can be changed within the parameters of health services.

Other preventive measures in primary care are, of necessity, indirect; that is, they are aimed at risk factors that are one step removed from health outcomes and whose modification involves changes in behaviours that are strongly socially patterned. For example, screening for cardiovascular disease identifies individuals at high risk of developing coronary heart disease, taking into account several risk factors – including hypertension, smoking and dietary habits – that are rooted in the norms and lifestyles of particular social groups. Prevention in these circumstances is aimed at changing behaviours and managing symptoms such as hypertension, rather than having a direct impact on outcomes. Very little is still known about 'what works' to improve the health of disadvantaged groups and reduce health inequalities in such circumstances. Although the research and policy agendas have moved on from understanding health inequalities to tackling them, there remains relatively little systematic evidence of what leads certain social groups to take greater health risks than others, even when they are aware of the risks that they are taking.

Without such understanding, as Birch (1999) indicates, attempts to enable these groups to change behaviours may have little effect. This accords with the view that 'high-risk' prevention strategies – identifying high-risk susceptible individuals to offer them some individual protection – are often behaviourally inappropriate (Rose 1985). Lifestyle characteristics, such as eating habits, smoking and exercise, are tightly bound by social norms that determine how we interact with our peers; a 'healthier' lifestyle may transgress such norms. Townsend *et al.* (1994) powerfully demonstrated this by showing how health education messages had a big impact on smoking cessation for higher social classes, but for social classes IV and V had little effect. National policies to raise the price of cigarettes have in the past had more impact on smoking cessation for lower socio-economic groups, but this reflects a different preventive strategy, one that aims to control the causes of disease for the population as a whole, rather than targeting those in 'high-risk' groups (Rose 1985). There is still much to be learnt about strategies for preventing ill health and their impact on health inequality in relation to conditions that depend on changing behaviour.

Inevitably, PCTs will be faced with deciding what are the most important inequalities that exist in their localities that need to be (and can be) addressed in the primary health context. This decision will almost certainly involve trade-offs between equity and equality, as well as trade-offs between equality and efficiency (Williams 2001). As has been emphasized throughout this chapter, health inequalities, especially those caused by health-related behaviours, may well arise in relation to ethnicity, gender and age as well as socio-economic status. The question as to whether they are avoidable, given appropriate primary care, is but one stage of the decision-making process. For instance, inequalities in life expectancy between men and women are marked, but are generally dismissed as unimportant because they are likely to be biologically based and thus not subject to change via medical intervention. Excess mortality for males is, however, largely due to behaviours and lifestyles that are socially patterned by gender. Such inequality is thus potentially avoidable, given effective preventive medicine, but is its reduction a higher priority than other inequalities, such as those associated with poverty, age and ethnicity?

Moreover, if inequality is reduced, does it matter how this is achieved? Gender inequalities in smoking behaviour have narrowed because there has been a lower rate of smoking cessation for women compared with men. Narrowing inequality in the coverage of measles, mumps and rubella immunizations in affluent and deprived areas in the latter half of the 1990s occurred because coverage fell faster in affluent areas. Are these desirable outcomes? Currently there is no clear moral, ethical or financial guidance on which to base local priorities about which inequalities to tackle in situations where 'equality/equality trade-offs' are necessary. Nor is there clear guidance on how to tackle them, particularly where improving the health of particular disadvantaged groups calls for specific interventions that will not necessarily benefit the whole of the population.

Conclusions

Perhaps a major achievement of the current government is to have situated health inequalities as a central plank in health policy. However, the role of PCTs in reducing inequality is diffuse and lacks strategic direction. There is a danger that, rather than attempting to tackle the confusion associated with this agenda, PCTs will simply relegate health inequalities to the bottom of their pile of priorities. This is evident in the recent official consultation document on 'tackling health inequalities' (Department of Health 2002). The document assigned a pivotal role to PCTs in drawing the NHS into the health inequalities agenda. However, 'getting it right' on the ground was more difficult, not least because of the risk of overlapping programmes and initiatives. Moreover, PCTs perceived health inequalities as a relatively low priority, were giving preference to secondary care in their plans, and felt they were already overburdened in deprived areas (Department of Health 2002).

There has been concern in some quarters (Birch 1999) that in outlining the potential role of PCTs in reducing health inequality, the government has relied too heavily on recommendations in the Acheson Report, *Independent Inquiry into Inequalities in Health* (Acheson et al. 1998; Williams and Illsley 2001). The Acheson Report identified the distribution of income as one of the 'upstream' structural factors associated with inequalities in health. However, as Birch (1999) has pointed out, the recommendations of the Acheson Report are based on the naive argument that policies which increase the income of the poorest are likely to improve their living standards, such as nutrition and heating, and so lead to improvements in health. But as discussed earlier, there is little evidence that improving standards of living will have this direct effect on health; certainly programmes of 'welfare to work' have no such demonstrable effect (O'Campo and Rojas-Smith 1998; Baker et al. 1999; Kncipp 2000). Yet PCTs are urged to engage in activities that address areas as diverse as housing, transport and community development to reduce health inequality (Gillam and Banks-Smith 2001). Apart from the challenge of integrated planning between PCTs and local authorities (see Chapter 12), it is unclear what effective role PCTs have to play in regeneration programmes. Indeed, of the 105 objectives outlined in the National Strategy for Neighbourhood Renewal, only nine were related to health services (Gillam and Banks-Smith 2001).

From vision to reality

The national health inequality targets provide a general focus of appropriate activities for PCTs; these include reducing inequalities in infant mortality, life expectancy, child poverty, rates of smoking and conceptions among women under the age of 18 between the most deprived populations and the population as a whole (Department of Health 2000). Nevertheless, the generality of these targets may be inappropriate for the purposes of local decision-making. Inequalities at the local level may arise from different population mixes and more or less severe health problems relating, for example, to ethnicity, age, socio-economic status, rural or urban conditions and so on (Petticrew and MacIntyre 2001). Thus the inequalities that matter most will vary from one locality to another. It may also be necessary to focus public policy not just on pursuing national targets, but on creating conditions in which local agencies can tackle those inequalities that they consider particularly important.

The public health function is essential for PCTs if they are to tackle health inequalities and the extent to which they are able to increase their capacity in public health will be one determinant of their success. The eclectic history of public health means that it is well placed to take on board evidence from a wide variety of disciplines in deciding on appropriate local strategies and determining which inequalities are important and what can realistically be done centrally and locally to reduce them.

References

Acheson, D., Barker, D., Chambers, J. *et al.* (1998) *Independent Inquiry into Inequalities in Health: Report.* London: The Stationery Office.

Baker, D. and Hann, M. (2001) General practitioner services in Primary Care Groups in England: is there inequity between service availability and population need?, *Health and Place,* 7(2): 67–74.

Baker, D. and Middleton, E. (2003) Cervical screening and health inequality in England in the 1990s, *Journal of Epidemiology and Community Health,* 57(6): 417–23.

Baker, D., Klein, R. and Carter, R. (1994) The impact of the 1990 contract for general practitioners on night visiting, *Journal of General Practice,* 44(379): 68–71.

Baker, D., North, K. and ALSPAC Study Team (1999) Does employment improve the health of lone mothers?, *Social Science and Medicine,* 49(1): 121–31.

Baker, D., Mead, N. and Campbell, S. (2002) Inequalities in morbidity and consulting behaviour for socially vulnerable groups, *British Journal of General Practice,* 52(475): 124–30.

Benzeval, M. and Judge, K. (1996) Access to healthcare in England: continuing inequalities in the distribution of GPs, *Journal of Public Health Medicine,* 18(1): 33–40.

Birch, S. (1999) The 39 steps: the mystery of health inequalities in the UK, *Health Economics,* 8(4): 301–8.

Carr-Hill, R. and Sheldon, T. (1991) Designing a deprivation payment for general practitioners: the UPA(8) wonderland, *British Medical Journal,* 302(6773): 393–6.

Carr-Hill, R. and Sheldon, T. (1992) Rationality and the use of formulae in the allocation of resources to health care, *Journal of Public Health Medicine*, 14(2): 117–26.

Carr-Hill, R., Rice, N. and Smith, P. (1998) *Towards Locally Based Resource Allocation in the NHS*, Discussion Paper 59. York: Centre for Health Economics, University of York.

Charlton, J.R.H and Velez, R. (1986) Some international comparisons of mortality amenable to medical intervention, *British Medical Journal*, 292(6516): 295–301.

Culyer, A. (2001) Equity – some theory and its implications, *Journal of Medical Ethics*, 27(4): 275–83.

Daniels, N., Light, D. and Caplan, R. (1996) *Benchmarks of Fairness for Health Care Reform*. Oxford: Oxford University Press.

Department of Health (2000) *The NHS Plan: A Plan for Investment, a Plan for Reform*. London: The Stationery Office.

Department of Health (2002) *Tackling Health Inequalities: The Results of the Consultation Exercise*. London: Department of Health.

Dibben, C., Sims, A. and Noble, M. (2001) *Health Poverty Index Scoping Project*. Oxford: University of Oxford and South East Public Health Observatory.

Gillam, S. and Banks-Smith, J. (2001) Can primary care groups and trusts improve health?, *British Medical Journal*, 323(7304): 89–92.

Gravelle, H. and Sutton, M. (2001) Inequality in the geographical distribution of general practitioners in England and Wales 1974–1995, *Journal of Health Services Research and Policy*, 6(1): 6–13.

Gwatkin, D. (2000) Health inequalities and the health of the poor. What do we know? What can we do? *Bulletin of the World Health Organization*, 78(1): 3–18.

Hann, M. and Baker, D. (2002) *Population Need and the Provision of Primary Care in South Derbyshire*. Manchester: The University of Manchester.

Hart, N. (1986) Inequalities in health: the individual versus the environment, *Journal of the Royal Statistical Society Series A*, 149(3): 228–46.

Ibbotson, T., Wyke, S., McEwen, J., Macintyre, S. and Kelly, M. (1996) Uptake of cervical screening in general practice: effect of practice organization, structure and deprivation, *Journal of Medical Screening*, 3(1): 35–9.

Jarman, B. (1983) Identification of underprivileged areas, *British Medical Journal*, 286(6379): 1705–9.

Jarman, B. (1991) Jarman Index, *British Medical Journal*, 302(6782): 961–2.

Kneipp, S. (2000) The health of women in transition from welfare to employment, *Western Journal of Nursing Research*, 22(6): 656–82.

Kunst, A.E., Groenhof, F., Mackenbach, J. and EU Working Group on Socio-economic Inequalities in Health (1998) Occupational class and cause specific mortality in middle aged men in 11 European countries, *British Medical Journal*, 316(7145): 1636–42.

Leese, B. and Bosanquet, N. (1995) Change in general practice and its effects on service provision in areas with different socioeconomic characteristics, *British Medical Journal*, 311(7004): 546–50.

Le Grand, J. (1982) *The Strategy of Equality. Redistribution and the Social Services.* London: George Allen & Unwin.

Lynch, M. (1995) Effect of practice and patient population characteristics on the uptake of childhood immunizations, *British Journal of General Practice*, 45(393): 205–8.

Mackenbach, J. (1996) The contribution of medical care to mortality decline: McKeown revisited, *Journal of Clinical Epidemiology*, 49: 1207–13.

Majeed, A., Cook, D., Anderson, H.R. *et al.* (1994) Using patient and general practice characteristics to explain variation in cervical smear uptake rates, *British Medical Journal*, 308(6939): 1272–6.

Marchand, S., Wikler, D. and Landesman, B. (1998) Class, health, and justice, *The Milbank Quarterly*, 76(3): 449–67.

McKeown, T. (1979) *The Role of Medicine: Dream, Mirage or Nemesis?* Oxford: Blackwell.

McPherson, K., Wennberg, J., Hovind, O. and Clifford, P. (1982) Small area variation in the use of common surgical procedures: an international comparison of New England, England and Norway, *New England Journal of Medicine*, 307(21): 1310–14.

Middleton, E. and Baker, D. (2003) Comparison of social distribution of immunisation with measles, mumps and rubella vaccine, England, 1991–2001, *British Medical Journal*, 326(7394): 854.

Mooney, G. (1983) Equity in health care: confronting the confusion, *Effective Health Care*, 1(4): 179–84.

O'Campo, P. and Rojas-Smith, L. (1998) Welfare reforms and women's health: review of the literature and implications for state policy, *Journal of Public Health Policy*, 19(4): 420–46.

Olsen, J. (1997) Theories of justice and their implications for priority setting in health care, *Journal of Health Economics*, 16(6): 625–9.

Petticrew, M. and MacIntyre, S. (2001) What do we know about the effectiveness, and cost effectiveness of measures to reduce inequalities in health?, in A. Oliver, R. Cookson and D. McDaid (eds) *The Issues Panel for Equity in Health*. London: The Nuffield Trust.

Reading, R., Colver, A., Openshaw, S. and Jarvis, S. (1994) Do interventions that improve immunization uptake also reduce social inequalities in uptake, *British Medical Journal*, 308(6937): 1142–4.

Rose, G. (1985) Sick individuals and sick populations, *International Journal of Epidemiology*, 14(1): 32–9.

Rutstein, D., Berenberg, W., Chalmers, T. *et al.* (1976) Measuring the quality of medical care, *New England Journal of Medicine*, 294(11): 582–8.

Secretary of State for Health (1997) *The New NHS: Modern, Dependable*, Cm. 3807. London: The Stationery Office.

Sen, A. (1982) *Choice, Welfare and Measurement.* Oxford: Blackwell.

Senior, M.L. (1991) Deprivation payments to general practitioners: not what the doctor ordered, *Environment and Planning C: Government and Policy*, 9(1): 74–94.

Sheldon, T., Smith, G. and Bevan, G. (1993) Weighting in the dark: resource allocation in the new NHS, *British Medical Journal*, 306(6881): 835–9.

Szreter, S. (1988) The importance of social intervention in Britain's mortality decline *c*. 1850–1914: a re-interpretation of the role of public health, *Social History of Medicine*, 1(1): 1–37.

Tobias, M. and Jackson, G. (2001) Avoidable mortality in New Zealand, 1981–7, *Australian and New Zealand Journal of Public Health*, 25(1): 12–19.

Townsend, J. (1995) The burden of smoking, in M. Benezeval, K. Judge and M. Whitehead (eds) *Tackling Inequalities in Health*. London: King's Fund.

Townsend, J., Roderick, P. and Cooper, J. (1994) Cigarette smoking by socio-economic group, sex and age: effects of price, income and health publicity, *British Medical Journal*, 309(6959): 923–7.

Tudor Hart, J. (1971) The inverse care law, *Lancet*, 1(7696): 405–12.

van Doorslaer, E., Wagstaff, A., van der Burg, H. *et al.* (2000) Equity in the delivery of health care in Europe and the US, *Journal of Health Economics*, 19(5): 553–83.

Victora, C., Vaughan, J., Barros, F., Silva, A. and Tomasi, E. (2000) Explaining trends in inequities: evidence from Brazilian child health studies, *Lancet*, 356: 1093–8.

Williams, A. (2001) Equity and cost effectiveness: a short note, in A. Oliver, R. Cookson and D. McDaid (eds) *The Issues Panel for Equity in Health*. London: The Nuffield Trust.

Williams, A. and Illsley, R. (2001) Equity and health: an introductory preamble, in A. Oliver, R. Cookson and D. McDaid (eds) *The Issue Panel for Equity in Health*. London: The Nuffield Trust.

5 The new institutional structures

Risks to the doctor–patient relationship

Bronwyn Croxson, Brian Ferguson and Justin Keen

Introduction

Since the internal market was introduced in the early 1990s, there has been a formal distinction between the commissioning and provision of health care services within the National Health Service (NHS). However, one of the organizational features of the internal market was the introduction of fundholding that allowed general practitioners (GPs) in practices that joined the scheme to act as purchasers as well as providers of services. Moreover, other GPs, through alternative mechanisms such as commissioning groups, total purchasing pilot schemes and other less formal consultation processes, were given an input into the purchasing role, since they were consulted about purchasing decisions by health authorities. There was debate about the extent to which any tensions between the two roles were important, particularly in jeopardizing the quality of patient care, but there is little evidence that it affected the quality of care provided by GPs.

The reforms outlined by the Labour government in its 1997 White Paper *The New NHS: Modern, Dependable* (Secretary of State for Health 1997) included a new organizational form, primary care groups (PCGs), which, as discussed in Chapter 1 and Chapter 6, have now been superseded by primary care trusts (PCTs). These organizations also combine the two roles. The commissioning role is central to PCTs, with 75 per cent of the total NHS budget being allocated to them. In addition, many PCTs have a substantial providing role, including community health services as well as primary care. It is also intended that budget holding should give them an incentive to expand the range of services they provide 'in-house' if they can do so cost-effectively.

As described in Chapters 1 and 6, PCTs comprise local groups of GPs, with a central management team. Within this structure, most GPs remain independent contractors, with their practices in effect continuing to be run as small businesses. Although local GPs are integral to the management arrangements of PCTs, the viability of their practices and the services they provide to their own patients may therefore remain their prime concern.

Integrating the commissioning and providing roles within one organization may generate at least two types of conflict of interest for health care professionals, particularly GPs. The first arises if there is conflict between a GP's interests on the one hand and the health of his or her patients on the other. The phenomenon of supplier-induced demand is one manifestation of this type of conflict, which is further influenced by the behaviour of NHS and other organizations that affect traditional patterns of referral and service provision. The second conflict of interest arises if GPs are expected to assume responsibility for both the health of individual patients and the cost-effective allocation of resources across a local population. In this case, a conflict of interest arises if the health of one individual patient can be improved only at the expense of another's health, as must occur when allocating scarce resources. This type of conflict is inevitable, since the responsibility for processing the 'tough choices' facing the NHS has now been delegated to PCTs and their constituent GPs.

This chapter shows how an important part of economic theory, principal–agent theory, can be used in an accessible way to analyse these conflicts and to inform policy analysis. Depending on the incentive structure, supplier-induced demand may result from an imperfect principal–agent relationship. By vertically integrating commissioning and providing, the institutional arrangements governing PCTs increase the scope for opportunistic supplier-induced demand. They also create a situation in which there are 'multiple principals'. Whether the potential for opportunism and confused responsibilities is realized depends on the effect of the overall governance structure of primary care, including professional ethics as well as regulations and incentives.

Addressing this issue is further complicated by major changes in GPs' employment contracts (see Chapter 1), notably the introduction of personal medical services contracts, some forms of which allow GPs to work as salaried employees of the NHS, and the new general medical services contract. The details of the new general medical services contract are consistent with the general arguments set out below.

In the next section, we discuss the application of principal–agent theory in this context, and the way in which PCTs embody vertical integration between purchasing and providing. We then consider the reasons why GPs might seek vertical integration. In the final sections, we discuss incentive structures and suggest a way forward for designing a regulatory framework for primary care. We conclude that a framework designed to promote accountability should accompany changes to the institutional environment, if the relationship between GPs and patients is to be properly protected. This has parallels with changes in the regulation of private industry, where the government has strengthened consumer protection in specific sectors such as financial services (Financial Services and Markets Bill 1999) and invested substantial general powers in the Office of Fair Trading and the Competition Commission (Pickersgill 1999).

Principal–agent models

The relationship between patients and GPs is often analysed as an example of a generic class of economic relationships, principal–agent relationships (Propper 1995). A principal–agent relationship exists if one person, a principal, delegates an activity affecting the principal's well being to another, the agent. Patients are assumed to want to delegate decisions about health care to their doctor (their agent) if there is a high cost to acquiring relevant information or if they are anxious or unable to take a decision themselves (Mooney and Ryan 1993). Problems arise if the agent's and principal's objectives differ, since this means the agent will not necessarily act in the interests of the principal. There is a substantial economics literature analysing the nature of principal–agent relationships, particularly the circumstances necessary to ensure that agents do act in the interests of principals when they have different objectives. In general, aligning the interests of the two parties depends on being able to give agents an incentive to act in the interests of their principal and/or on the principal being able to monitor the agent without incurring unreasonable costs (Arrow 1986).

In the context of health care, patients and their doctors share at least some relevant objectives. There is evidence that GPs seek to improve patient health and welfare. There is, however, also evidence that objectives may diverge, because GPs' desire for leisure time, income and personal autonomy may sometimes conflict with delivering patient care (Scott 1997). For example, GPs may trade off time spent with patients against time spent with their own families. In this case, the principal–agent relationship is said to be imperfect, with outcomes that do not necessarily reflect principals' interests.

Problems resulting from divergent objectives can be mitigated if principals monitor agents. Monitoring is costly in health care, however, since there is usually a difference in the information available to patients and to GPs (termed 'asymmetric information'). Doctors have specialized knowledge and expertise and it will generally be costly for patients to monitor GPs' actions and arrive at informed assessments of the advice they are offered. These costs are compounded by the inexact nature of medical science, which makes it difficult to establish whether an adverse clinical outcome results from negligence by either party or is simply an 'act of God' (Mooney and Ryan 1993).

The prevailing institutional structure affects both the extent of any divergence between the objectives of GPs and patients and the costs of monitoring GPs. The patient is not alone in monitoring and assessing the work of GPs, as there are various institutional arrangements governing the patient–GP relationship. These include the regulations covering GPs' contractual obligations, whether under the traditional general medical services or the new personal medical services contract (see Chapter 1); arrangements for peer review; and professional ethics. The relationship is also affected by the incentives associated with the rules for remuneration of GPs (Donaldson and Gerard 1989). All of these institutional arrangements can be conceptualized as affecting the costs and benefits to GPs of different forms of behaviour. A change to the institutional arrangements, such as the introduction of a new general medical services contract, may for example alter GPs' preferred trade-offs between time spent at work and time spent with their families, by altering their assessment of the costs and benefits attached to each. Indeed, this is exactly what seems to have been happening during the 1990s, with GPs arguing that their workloads were too high and their representatives pressing the government to place upper limits on GPs' time commitments. The proposed new general medical services contract reflects this, placing clear limits on GPs' workload in a way that its predecessor did not. Changing institutional arrangements may also affect the costs of monitoring and assessing GP behaviour, since different structures will make the tasks more or less easy and therefore more or less costly.

This type of analysis, recognizing the role of institutional structures in influencing the behaviour of GPs as agents, echoes the work of public choice theorists, who have proposed models of the behaviour of senior public servants that are useful when analysing GP behaviour. Broadly, there are two public choice models. The first proposes that bureaucrats should maximize their departmental budgets, partly because this provides them with personal benefits such as higher salaries – budget-maximizing theories. The second proposes that they should be motivated to shape their departments to maximize the amount of 'interesting' work they do, such as policy analysis, rather than 'boring' administration – bureau-shaping theories (Dunleavy 1991; James 1995). In a similar vein, GPs may act as either budget maximizers or as bureau shapers. That is, they may have incentives to pursue objectives that are not related to patient welfare, but instead seek to maximize their personal or group practice income, or to shape their work practices to suit their own preferences.

By combining commissioning and providing, PCTs give GPs greater latitude to pursue their own objectives. Moreover, within PCTs, GPs are required to pursue activities that are not directly related to the welfare of their patients, such as responsibility for resource allocation. In other words, the new structures place greater pressure on the patient–GP principal–agent relationship, by requiring that GPs pursue objectives not directly related to patient care. We discuss these issues below, after introducing empirical evidence about the impact on the patient–GP relationship of two earlier organizational forms that also integrated commissioning and providing.

Vertically integrating commissioning and providing

Vertical integration occurs when the consecutive activities required to deliver a particular service are combined within the same organization. The NHS internal market introduced vertical integration between the commissioning and provision of some primary care services, through GP fundholding and total purchasing. Under GP fundholding, GPs were able to purchase some community health services and a limited set of (mainly elective) hospital procedures, and they controlled their prescribing budgets. In total purchasing, which was a voluntary extension of fundholding, groups of general practices jointly controlled a budget, which could in principle be used to commission all hospital and community health services for their registered populations (Mays *et al.* 1998). As the first arrangements explicitly to vertically integrate purchasing and providing in primary care, they are a useful source of empirical information about the effects of changing the institutional arrangements surrounding GPs.

There is evidence that fundholders changed their activity in specific areas, compared with both their own past behaviour and the behaviour of other GPs, for example in their prescribing practices and in the temporal pattern of some elective activity (Coulter and Bradlow 1993; Whynes *et al.* 1995; Croxson *et al.* 2001). However, there is no evidence of any change in the level or pattern of emergency activity (Audit Commission 1996; Toth *et al.* 1997; Croxson *et al.* 2001). Moreover, Ellwood (1997) found that GP fundholders did sometimes change the nature and volume of services they offered, but that they did not respond to changes in price, and did not make the savings that would have been possible by 'shopping around' locally.

The evidence from the evaluation of total purchasing is that most projects focused their commissioning efforts on selected services (Goodwin *et al.* 1999; Malbon *et al.* 1999). A number were able to change the patterns of specific services within primary care settings (for example, by employing a counsellor to work in a practice), while a few achieved changes in service delivery in specific areas such as services for the mentally ill. There was, however, little fundamental change, and the changes that did occur concentrated on improving processes (for example, generating information that could be used for commissioning decisions) rather than service provision. There is little evidence that patient outcomes were substantially affected and it is notable that one-third of total purchasing sites had dropped out after 2 years.

One feature of both fundholding and total purchasing was that projects were able to retain any financial savings made during a particular year. This arrangement was designed to encourage cost-effective practice, but it also contained incentives for inappropriate cost-saving behaviour. There was, for example, an incentive for 'cream-skimming' of patient lists, with GPs retaining only low-risk, low-cost patients. There is no evidence that fundholders did engage in cream-skimming, possibly because they did not have to fund the care of high-cost patients. It is not clear whether this behaviour occurred in the total purchasing projects, but it is unlikely (Malbon *et al.* 1999).

Crucially, the doctor–patient relationship does not appear to have been systematically affected, either positively or negatively, by GP fundholding or total purchasing, at least according to this evidence. Therefore, a key issue is whether the additional flexibility and responsibility given to GPs in PCTs threatens the principal–agent relationship in a way that fundholding did not. We first outline the nature of the vertical integration in PCTs, then the factors that are likely to protect patients, before considering the way in which the new structures could have deleterious consequences for patients.

Vertical integration in primary care trusts

Primary care trusts expand the ability of GPs to commission 'packages' of health care that combine a range of different services. Each PCT has a unified budget (see Chapter 6) and is responsible for commissioning all NHS services required by its patients, and also non-NHS services where deemed appropriate. Hence there is vertical integration between commissioning on the one hand and delivery of primary care and community services on the other. New legislation further extends the potential for PCTs to provide social, as well as health, services. For example, Section 31 of the Health Act 1999 allows for the creation of new organizations, which sit between the NHS and social services, and are able to combine health and social care services (see Chapter 12). Primary care trusts now also have the powers to purchase nursing home care.

The evidence outlined above suggests that fundholding and total purchasing were not accompanied by significant changes in GP behaviour. However, PCTs have greater commissioning and providing roles, meaning that GPs will have greater flexibility and responsibility. A key issue is whether these pose a threat to the principal–agent relationship in a way that fundholding did not.

One factor likely to protect patients is the impact on individual GPs' behaviour of peer review by other GPs in the PCT. However, the effect of this protection is likely to be weakened if PCTs experience coordination problems. Primary care trusts combine large numbers of previously separate GPs from different general practices, as well as other professional groups. They are therefore likely to experience considerable internal coordination problems. These problems arise because PCTs are new entities responsible for commissioning and providing new combinations of health (and social) services, and they are comprised of individuals with naturally diverse backgrounds and values. Coordination problems are likely to impede PCTs' ability to act as organizations, giving some parts of the organization only limited control over the actions of others, and may allow individual GPs to follow their own interests, possibly at the expense of wider PCT objectives (see Chapter 2).

It is difficult to analyse the impact of the flexibility offered by vertical integration on the agency relationship itself. General practitioners may or may not be more inclined to follow their own interests than the interests of their patients. However, it is certainly the case that greater devolution of budgetary control will increase the scope for this, increasing as it does the ability of GPs to shape their behaviours in ways that reflect their own needs and those of their practices. Some additional protection is offered through monitoring by strategic health authorities against annual accountability agreements and health improvement plans. But the effectiveness of this depends on whether the new strategic health authorities regulate on behalf of patients or, as implied in new policies, the local population. As will be discussed in the next section, the interests of the two groups may well diverge.

The ability of a PCT to commission services in ways that respond to new and changing needs may be limited because some parts of the organization will have only limited control over the actions of others. In the short term, a lack of coordination might protect the agency relationship between individual patients and some GPs, but this is equivalent to free-riding by individual GPs and, with cash-limited budgets, can be sustained in the long run only at the expense of other GPs and their patients. This trade-off between the services that different GPs provide has until now been disguised because it has not been made explicit within NHS budgets. At the very least, PCTs will face these trade-offs more directly in the future.

Multiple principals

The fundamental safeguard to the doctor–patient principal–agent relationship is professional ethics – a commitment by doctors to act in the best clinical interests of the people in front of them. The ethical duty of doctors, absorbed during their training and practice, is a bulwark against either deliberate opportunism or simply following their own personal objectives. These might be manifest as a desire to treat only interesting cases, to have additional leisure time or to spend income on practice facilities.

As we have argued, however, the new institutional arrangements set up conflicting incentives for GPs. On the one hand, their ethical principles are oriented towards acting as the agents of individual patients; on the other, they are required to ration resources, as if they are the agents of taxpayers. Sometimes the conflict between acting in the best interests of patients and the rational allocation of resources arises from external regulations. One example is the requirement to achieve the target of ensuring that patients suspected of having cancer are seen by a specialist within 2 weeks of referral (NHS Executive 1999a), which inevitably places a burden on GPs to balance the risk of not referring against the budgetary impact of referring all cases that could potentially benefit. Although this raises some complex issues about GPs' attitudes to risk, it is a clear example of the wider responsibility that GPs now have within their PCTs to undertake what are, in effect, explicit rationing decisions.

Several economists have recognized that health care comprises a complex set of overlapping agency relationships (Propper 1995), and that in practice GPs do take into account considerations wider than those arising directly from the GP–patient relationship (for example, health promotion activities within practices). However, the new structure raises the question of whose interests GPs should represent. Although principal–agent theory is built on the assumption that the principal and agent can be identified, there are several contexts where the identity of a principal is unclear. This has been recognized in recent theoretical work that seeks to extend principal–agent theory to incorporate multi-agent or multi-principal models (Varian 1990; Itoh 1994; Krepps and Caves 1994). It has also been recognized by Smith and Wright (1994) in the context of social care, where they argue that there may be conflict between the interests of carers and patients, and it is not clear whose interests social care providers should follow.

In their first capacity, as the agents of patients, GPs are effectively advocates for individuals, ensuring that each individual has access to the best available services. This role is certainly visible in the new structure. Indeed, the 1997 White Paper states that the increased purchasing power and greater flexibility offered by a unified budget 'will give GPs the maximum choice about the treatment option that best suits individual patients, free from the constraints imposed by artificially distinct budget headings' (Secretary of State for Health 1997: 70).

With a unified budget, however, PCTs also have responsibility for cost-effective resource allocation across an entire population. General practitioners have traditionally acted as gatekeepers to secondary care, since non-emergency patients have always needed a GP referral to see a specialist. However, GPs were not under a binding budget constraint and so did not face the conflicting objectives they are now confronted with in PCTs. The responsibility for resource allocation has been extended, since the new vertically integrated structure requires that PCTs commission all services, effectively having to make rationing decisions across their patient populations. Moreover, notwithstanding their independent contractor status, GPs are now formally part of the NHS organizational chart in a way that they were not before. The PCTs to which they belong are accountable through strategic health authorities to the Department of Health and ultimately to the Secretary of State (NHS Executive 1999b).

This may generate a fundamental contradiction for GPs. On the one hand, GPs have a responsibility to do the best they can for individual patients, while on the other, they may have to deny a specific individual access to care if it is not consistent with priorities agreed by the PCT. This tension has been recognized in the literature, both in the context of health care (Mooney and Ryan 1993) and in the more general context of the changing relationship between professionals and the state, with professionals increasingly under pressure to become the agents of the state (and therefore also of taxpayers) rather than of their direct clients (Ferlie *et al.* 1996). The tension has not, however, been recognized in the context of governing PCTs. The new PCTs may work effectively only if GPs abandon their traditional role as agents of individual patients, a role that grows out of their professional ethics. This means that if they do accept their new role, an unintended consequence might be the undermining of these ethics, in which case the traditional protection for individual patients will be eroded.

The new contracts

It has become increasingly clear over the last few years that GPs' contract to provide general medical services to their registered patients, whose main features have been in place since the founding of the NHS in 1948, has not been working to anyone's advantage. The contract is written in very general terms, effectively requiring GPs to see anyone who comes to a practice. The boundaries of GPs' work were not defined; general practice was what GPs did. The original spirit of the contract, wherein GPs were the first port of call for most people, had over time come to mean that GPs found themselves dealing with an ever-wider range of problems and workloads that were simply becoming too great. There was also an underlying trend in the reducing willingness of GPs to work flat out. More wanted to work part-time and to have what they believed to be a reasonable amount of leisure time. Paying GPs more would result in better-off but still exhausted GPs.

Successive governments have presided over the increasing problems with GPs and arguably contributed to these problems, for example by imposing ever-greater administrative loads. Equally though, both Conservative and (especially) Labour governments have become frustrated. It has been difficult to get GPs to work in unpopular localities where the health needs were greatest or to persuade GPs to be more 'patient-friendly', for example by holding surgeries in the early morning and the evening to fit in with their patients' longer working days. There have been two important policy responses to these problems that involve new contracts of employment: personal medical services contracts and the new general medical services contract.

Personal medical services contracts

By 2003, almost 25 per cent of GPs were working under personal medical services (PMS) contracts. These contracts take different forms, but the key point here is that GPs can opt to work as salaried employees of the NHS rather than as independent contractors, and work only for a specified number of hours. Many PMS schemes have been set up in localities where there is a history of difficulties in attracting GPs, such as parts of southeast London and inner-city Birmingham. Personal medical services contracts were initially negotiated with health authorities, but are now managed by PCTs.

The evaluation of the first wave of PMS pilots (PMS National Evaluation Team 2002) suggests that the GPs involved were making an explicit trade-off between work and leisure time and opted for more of the latter, to the extent that on average in 1999 GPs working on a PMS contract earned less than GP principals on general medical services (GMS) contracts. This difference was to some extent offset by a constant income (which can fluctuate under GMS) and benefits such as easier access to educational leave and better maternity leave. It appears that the GPs who are attracted to PMS fit the bureau-shaping public choice model, since they appear to have been seeking the freedom to remodel their work practices, rather than the budget-maximizing model.

The PMS contract removes some of the potential for conflict noted above, since the incentives for supplier-induced demand are minimized. Indeed, since the number of GPs in some deprived areas has been increased (and the government is achieving at least one of its objectives), it could be argued that on balance PMS could be working in the interests of patients in general, thereby squaring the circle of serving the needs of both individuals and populations.

General medical services contract

It is still too early to comment on the new GMS contract (BMA General Practice Committee 2002) in any detail. However, it is worth noting that the proposals have characteristics in common with PMS contracts; GPs' workload will in future be specified in more detail and there will be an upper limit to their workload. There will also be considerable additional earnings potential for delivering high-quality care, so that GPs may not have to make the same trade-offs as under PMS. They may in future be able both to earn more and have more leisure time, depending on how effectively they balance the trade-off between workload and the quality of care provided.

Similarly, it is simply too early to say how far the new contracts might exacerbate or ameliorate the conflicts of interest outlined above. One might speculate that they will help to avoid problems, because the contracts help to emphasize the separate roles of commissioning and provision. Rather less positively, having GPs' input to commissioning may simply lead to PMS or GMS contracts that are loaded in favour of GPs, and the potential problems noted will not be addressed.

Conclusions: implications for accountability

The government's policies assume that strategic health authorities will act in the interests of their citizens, in terms of setting the broad strategic framework and being held to account for improvements in the health of their populations. Groups of GPs, meanwhile, are supposed to act on behalf of their 'natural communities' and undertake the commissioning role according to the direction provided by the strategic health authority, encompassed within annual accountability agreements, health improvement plans and other policy instruments.

These policies and legislation begin to specify how patients' interests will be balanced against the proper need to promote and maintain the motivation of service providers and, by emphasizing cooperation and partnership, implicitly address the need to align patient, GP and other stakeholder interests. If the rhetoric is successfully translated into practice, this might reinforce the ethical codes traditionally relied upon to safeguard the GP–patient relationship.

There are, however, reasons to be concerned that this will not happen. This paper has drawn on principal–agent theory to show that the structure of the 'new' NHS may place at risk the traditional safeguards of patient welfare. If PCTs are able to act primarily in their role as representatives of taxpayers, shaping their budgets accordingly, there is a danger that the agency relationship between patients and doctors will be undermined. If this results in incentives for constituent practices to select out patients, it will not be possible automatically to rely on professional ethics to avoid any adverse consequences. The policy implication is that an appropriate governance framework will need to be designed to address the problem of potentially conflicting incentives.

The framework governing PCTs needs to address the risk that GPs will seek to design or influence PCTs and other institutional structures to achieve non-clinical goals. The present government is placing emphasis on its clinical governance and performance management policies to resolve any such tensions. Professionals will be given latitude to deliver services locally in ways that they believe to be appropriate, but will be accountable to one another and more formally to the Department of Health. Although potential coordination problems may undermine the effectiveness of these safeguards, the creation of new forms of contract offers an additional mechanism for ensuring that GPs primarily pursue clinical goals.

In this connection, it is worth noting that the need to mediate between 'producer' and 'consumer' interests has already led to action by the current government in other areas. For example, it has invested considerable consumer protection powers in the Office of Fair Trading and in regulators such as the Financial Services Authority. Proposing that similar action is needed in the NHS, to promote accountability and protect users, is saying no more than that the government should consider aligning its policies in different sectors.

References

Arrow, K. (1986) Information and the market, in K.J. Arrow and M.D. Intriligator (eds) *Handbook of Mathematical Economics*. Amsterdam: North-Holland.

Audit Commission (1996) *What the Doctor Ordered: A Study of GP Fundholders in England and Wales*. London: The Stationery Office.

BMA General Practice Committee (2002) *Your Contract, Your Future: General Practice Contract and Explanatory Notes from the GPC*. London: BMA.

Coulter, A. and Bradlow, J. (1993) Effect of NHS reforms on general practitioners' referral patterns, *British Medical Journal*, 306(6875): 433–47.

Croxson, B., Propper, C. and Perkins, A. (2001) Do doctors respond to financial incentives? UK family doctors and the GP fundholder scheme, *Journal of Public Economics*, 79(2): 375–98.

Donaldson, C. and Gerard, K. (1989) Countering moral hazard within public and private health care systems: a review of recent evidence, *Journal of Social Policy*, 18(2): 235–51.

Dunleavy, P. (1991) *Democracy, Bureaucracy and Public Choice. Economic Explanations in Political Science*. Brighton: Harvester Wheatsheaf.

Ellwood, S. (1997) Have GPs been playing the market?, *The Fundholding Summary*, 5–8.

Ferlie, E., Ashburner, L., Fitzgerald, L. and Pettigrew, A. (1996) *The New Public Management in Action*. Oxford: Oxford University Press.

Goodwin, N., Abbott, S., Baxter, K. *et al.* (1999) *Analysis of Implications of Eleven Case Studies*. London: King's Fund.

Itoh, H. (1994) Job design, delegation and co-operation: a principal–agent analysis, *European Economic Review*, 38(3–4): 691–700.

James, O. (1995) Explaining the Next Steps in the Department of Social Security: the bureau-shaping model of central state re-organisation, *Political Studies*, 43(4): 614–29.

Krepps, M.B. and Caves, R.E. (1994) Bureaucrats and Indians – principal–agent relations and efficient management of tribal forest resources, *Journal of Economic Behaviour and Organisation*, 24(2): 133–51.

Malbon, G., Mays, N., Killoran, A., Wyke, S. and Goodwin, N. (1999) *What were the Achievements of Total Purchasing Pilots in their Second Year (1997/98) and how can they be Explained?* London: King's Fund.

Mays, N., Goodwin, N., Killoran, A. and Malbon, G. (1998) *Total Purchasing: A Step Towards Primary Care Groups.* London: King's Fund.

Mooney, G. and Ryan, M. (1993) Agency in health care: getting beyond first principles, *Journal of Health Economics*, 12(2): 125–35.

NHS Executive (1999a) *Cancer Waiting Times: Achieving the Two Week Target.* NHS Health Services Circular 1999/205. Leeds: NHS Executive.

NHS Executive (1999b) *Letter, 1999/098.* London: The Stationery Office.

Pickersgill, D. (1999) *The 1998 Competition Act Explained.* London: The Stationery Office.

PMS National Evaluation Team (2002) *Evaluation of First Wave NHS Personal Medical Services Pilots: Summaries of Findings from Four Research Projects.* London: Department of Health.

Propper, C. (1995) Agency and incentives in the NHS Internal Market, *Social Science and Medicine*, 40(12): 1683–90.

Scott, A. (1997) Designing incentives for GPs: A review of the literature on their preferences for pecuniary and non-pecuniary job characteristics. *HERU Discussion Paper.* Aberdeen: University of Aberdeen.

Secretary of State for Health (1997) *The New NHS: Modern, Dependable*, Cm. 3807. London: The Stationery Office.

Smith, K. and Wright, K. (1994) *Principals and Agents in Social Care: Who's on the Case and for Whom?* Discussion Paper. York: Centre for Health Economics, University of York.

Toth, B., Harvey, I. and Peters, T. (1997) Did the introduction of general practice fundholding change patterns of emergency admission to hospital?, *Journal of Health Service Research and Policy*, 2(2): 71–4.

Varian, H.R. (1990) Monitoring agents with other agents, *Journal of Institutional and Theoretical Economics*, 146: 153–74.

Whynes, D., Baines, D.L. and Tolley, K.H. (1995) GP fundholding and the costs of prescribing, *Journal of Public Health Medicine*, 17(3): 323–9.

PART 2
Inside primary care organizations

6 Organizational development and governance of primary care

Bernard Dowling, David Wilkin and Keri Smith

Introduction

Primary care has been given a central role in the government's plans for modernizing the National Health Service (NHS) (Department of Health 2001a). For primary care to be successful in driving the desired changes, the sector will require a strong and well-resourced organizational structure, including a workforce with the necessary skills and an appropriate budgetary framework. Primary care trusts (PCTs) will need to work alongside other organizations, both within and outside the NHS, that have been established for far longer. A fundamental question that arises from this issue is whether the early evidence suggests PCTs have the requisite capacity to meet these challenges.

Since its foundation in 1948, the NHS has lacked a unified organizational structure and system of governance. The original tripartite structure of hospitals, community health services and family practitioner services has been repeatedly reorganized (Ham 1992). But general practice and other family practitioner services have remained separately funded and organized, despite successive reforms to the bodies that administered these services, including executive councils, family practitioner committees and family health services authorities. Although the reforms in the early 1990s introducing an internal market to the NHS brought about radical changes in the funding and governance of hospital and community health services, they did little to change the funding, organization and governance of primary care. The centrepiece of the Labour government's 1997 White Paper for the NHS (Secretary of State for Health 1997) was the proposal to establish primary care groups (PCGs) and their anticipated progression to PCT status. Together with these organizational changes came significant revisions to the funding of primary care as a new budgetary framework was introduced.

These reforms built upon policies already promoted under the previous

Conservative administrations, including strengthening the role of primary care, shifting decision-making power closer to frontline health professionals, and promoting alternative ways of delivering primary and community health services. With control over a unified budget for health care, PCTs assumed responsibility for three core functions: commissioning health care; developing primary and community services; and improving health and reducing health inequalities for their registered populations (Department of Health 1998). Within a strong national framework of standards, regulation and inspection, the intention was to devolve responsibility for decisions about implementation to frontline primary care professionals, who were in the best position to understand the particular needs and circumstances of their local communities.

The creation of primary care groups and trusts (PCG/Ts) represented a radical reform of the organization and governance of the NHS that has been reinforced in subsequent policy guidance (Department of Health 2001a). The creation of a unified health care budget, the incorporation of primary care into mainstream NHS organization and governance, and the devolution of decision-making to networks of professional stakeholders were all radical changes to the way the NHS had been organized and governed during its first 50 years. The aim of this chapter is to review the experience of implementing these changes in organization and governance over the first 3 years of PCG/Ts. First, we describe the prescribed structure and governance arrangements of PCGs and PCTs. In the remainder of the chapter, we examine four important aspects of the changes in organization and governance: the representation of key stakeholders; the size, complexity and capacity of the organizations; the tensions between central control of the NHS and local autonomy; and the management of the new financial framework.

Organizational structures

The 1997 White Paper proposed four levels of primary care organization with increasing levels of autonomy (Secretary of State for Health 1997). Initially, all were accountable to the pre-April 2002 health authorities and subsequently to the newly created strategic health authorities (see Chapter 11 for a discussion of other potential lines of accountability). Subsequent policy documents (Secretary of State for Health 2000; Department of Health 2001a) elaborated and extended the scope of PCG/T responsibilities, including the significant proposal that PCTs would become responsible for managing and spending three-quarters of the total health care budget. Primary care groups at level 1 resembled the former locality commissioning groups and simply supported and advised the old health authorities. At level 2, PCGs took devolved responsibility for managing the health care budget but as subcommittees of the health authority (Secretary of State for Health 1997). All general practices and their registered patient populations were assigned to one of the 481 level 1 or 2 PCGs that were established in April 1999.

Levels 3 and 4 were to be freestanding trusts (PCTs), independent from but accountable to the health authorities. Level 3 PCTs would be responsible for commissioning hospital and community services, while level 4 PCTs would become providers of a range of community services as well as commissioning secondary and specialist services. The 1997 White Paper envisaged a process of developmental learning, through which PCGs would gradually progress to PCT status (Secretary of State for Health 1997). In practice, 30 PCGs became PCTs in 2000 after only a year; another 124 became PCTs in 2001; and the remainder became PCTs in 2002 as, following the implementation of *Shifting the Balance of Power* (Department of Health 2001a), the 95 old health authorities were abolished and replaced by 28 new strategic health authorities. This rapid and universal progression to PCT status by 2002 exceeded the government's target that all PCGs should become trusts by 2004 (Secretary of State for Health 2000). Virtually all PCTs have opted for level 4 trust status, in which they both commission and directly provide services. Primary care groups were thus a transitional stage on the road to full trust status.

As subcommittees of health authorities, PCGs were run by boards consisting of the chief executive, between four and seven general practitioners (GPs), one or two nurses, a social services representative, a health authority non-executive representative and one lay member (NHS Executive 1998). General practitioner board members, who were elected by all GPs from practices within the PCG, could hold a majority on the board as well as having the right to nominate the chair. Perhaps unsurprisingly, it was therefore common for PCG chairs to be GPs.

Governance arrangements for PCTs are similar in their emphasis on professional stakeholder representation, though they have a two-tier governance structure (Figure 6.1). The main policy and decision-making body of PCTs is the professional executive committee, similar in composition to the PCG board but with fewer GPs and more other health professionals. However, it should be noted that GPs remain the largest single professional group and that primary care professionals outnumber managers on the professional executive committee. The chair of the professional executive committee is elected from its professional members and is usually a GP. Executive committees are accountable to the PCT board: for complying with the broad legal framework, including NHS law and human rights; delivering the terms of annual accountability agreements (which should cover the local health improvement plan – see Chapter 10); and maintaining an effective strategic base (NHS Executive 1999).

In common with other NHS trusts, the PCT board has a majority of lay or non-executive members. It is responsible for overseeing the work of the

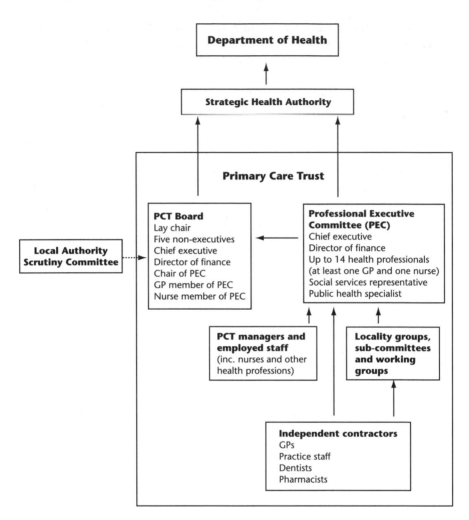

Figure 6.1   Organization and governance structure of primary care trusts.

professional executive committee and for ensuring probity, public involvement and public accountability. The boards of PCTs have three key roles: ensuring that the culture and direction of the organization complements the local community's needs; ensuring the organization maintains the best traditions of public service, including sustaining external relationships with the public, patients, local government and other partner organizations; and ensuring the PCT has clear processes for decision-making (NHS Executive 1999).

Much of the day-to-day work of the PCT is delegated to subcommittees or working groups of the professional executive committee and to managers and other staff employed directly by the PCT. Many larger PCTs have also begun to establish locality groups, with varying degrees of devolved responsibility for services in smaller areas within their boundaries. Primary care trusts are accountable to the new strategic health authorities that manage their performance; local authority overview and scrutiny committees (see Chapter 11) are intended to provide a further check on the activities of PCTs.

Stakeholders and governance

The creation of PCGs and PCTs was a conscious attempt to engage and represent local stakeholders, especially professionals, in the governance of the NHS. Arguably this had two intentions: to increase the scope for locality-sensitive decision-making; and to engage frontline professional staff in the management and governance of local NHS services, including the allocation and management of resources. The British Medical Association negotiated a potentially dominant and undoubtedly important role for GPs in PCGs (though their influence is less explicit in the governance of PCTs), as a condition of cooperation with and participation in the reforms by family doctors. However, this enhanced decision-making role for GPs also included major responsibilities for the establishment of new constraints on budgets and behaviour in the primary care sector, including the introduction of collective responsibility for the quality of care provided (see Chapter 7).

The PCG/T chairs recognized that the support of primary care professionals was fundamental to the success of their organizations. In 2002, according to the Tracker Survey (Wilkin *et al.* 2002), 97 per cent of board chairs rated the support of local GPs as important to the success of the PCG/T and 90 per cent rated the support of nurses as important. Chairs were also asked to estimate the actual support among local GPs and nurses for the organization. In the first year of the survey, 1999/2000, only 40 per cent of chairs felt that at least half of their local GPs were supportive. By the third year (2001/2), this had risen to 61 per cent. Although only a minority of GPs in any PCG/T were felt to be hostile, nevertheless in a quarter of PCG/Ts in 2001/2 the chairs reported that at least one in five of their GPs was negative or antagonistic.

The Tracker Survey examined PCG/T chairs' perceptions of the extent to which the interests of different stakeholder groups were represented in the decision-making processes of PCG boards and, from 2000/1 onwards, the professional executive committees of PCTs. Figure 6.2 shows the results of this comparison for GPs, nurses and local communities. In the opinion of PCG/T chairs, professional stakeholders' views were, by and large, successfully represented. However, by 2001/2, when all the primary care organizations had either become or were about to become PCTs, the proportion of chairs that felt professional stakeholders were well represented had declined slightly. In striking contrast, chairs were far less (and indeed decreasingly) confident that the views of the local community were well represented (Smith *et al.* 2002). This suggests that PCG/Ts may have been only partially successful in providing

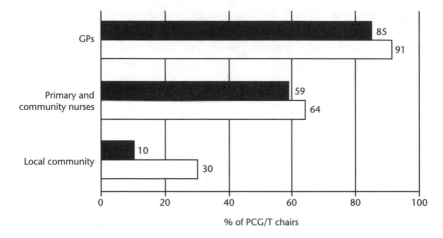

Figure 6.2 Percentages of stakeholders considered by PCG board chairs and PCT executive committee chairs to be well represented (2000/1 to 2001/2). Rated 4 or 5 on a 5-point scale from 1 'not at all' to 5 'very well'. ■, 2001/2; ❑, 2001/1. *Source*: Wilkin *et al.* (2002).

clear mechanisms for representing a wide range of local interests (this issue is discussed at greater length in Chapter 11).

The PCG/T chairs were asked to rate the amount of influence that different stakeholders had on the policies and priorities of the organization. In 2002, almost all (98 per cent) agreed that the principal officers and members of their governing bodies (the board chair, chief executive and chair of the PCT executive committee) held considerable influence (rated 4 or 5 on a 5-point scale), and 82 per cent said that the PCG board or PCT executive committee exercised considerable influence. However, despite the fact that PCG boards and PCT executive committees were intended to represent local primary care professionals, chairs were less confident that local GPs and nurses could really influence policy and priorities. Only 28 per cent of chairs rated local GPs and 11 per cent rated nurses as having considerable influence. But while this suggests that GPs had more influence than nurses, the most recent available evidence (Smith *et al.* 2002) indicates that nurses tend to be more supportive of PCG/Ts than GPs.

Moreover, the transition from PCG to PCT status appeared to lead to an increased concentration of power and influence in the officers of the organization and a corresponding decline in the influence of broader professional constituencies. In 2002, just 42 per cent of PCG board chairs rated their officers (such as the chair, chief executive, director of finance) as having very strong influence (rated 5 on a 5-point scale), compared with 70 per cent of PCT executive committee chairs. Conversely, only 12 per cent of PCG board chairs rated local GPs as having little or no influence (1 or 2 on a five-point scale), compared with 30 per cent of PCT executive committee chairs (Smith *et al*. 2002). This suggests the gap in influence between health professionals sitting on the governing body and their professional constituencies may have increased with the transition to trust status. However, the sustained levels of GP support for their primary care organization reported above suggests that the apparent increased discrepancy between the influence of GPs and managers, as PCGs became trusts, had not (yet) created serious tensions between them.

Despite the obligation placed on PCG/Ts to inform, consult and engage local communities in decision-making about health and health care, and despite the evidence of widespread efforts to fulfil this obligation, there is little evidence of success. Three-quarters of PCGs and PCTs (77 per cent) in 2002 had established public involvement working groups and employed a variety of methods for informing and consulting local communities. These included consulting local councillors (72 per cent), holding public meetings (70 per cent), consulting established patient groups (62 per cent), organizing focus groups or user forums (61 per cent) and analysing patient complaints (50 per cent). Nevertheless, only 18 per cent reported that their consultation processes were effective, with almost two-thirds believing that local people were still unaware of the existence of the organization and 84 per cent believing that local people did not know how to contribute to the processes of PCG/T decision-making (Smith *et al*. 2002). In PCTs the board, with its majority of lay members, could perhaps provide an alternative mechanism for involving the local community. However, the decision-making role of the PCT board is limited; its function is to oversee the work of the professional executive committee and ensure probity, rather than formulate policy and determine priorities itself. This limits the influence of lay PCT board members on decision-making, at a time when PCTs are also placing greater emphasis on national policies and targets than on local priorities (Smith *et al*. 2002). Further detailed evidence of the activities of PCTs to promote public participation and the possible reasons for their limited impact are discussed in Chapter 11.

Size, complexity and capacity

The 1997 White Paper proposed that PCGs should serve populations of around 100,000 people, enabling them to reflect and be responsive to the needs of local areas (Secretary of State for Health 1997). It also anticipated a process in which progress through the four levels of primary care organization would be based on developmental learning and the demonstration of a capacity to take on additional roles and responsibilities. The average population of the 481 PCGs established in April 1999 was approximately 100,000 (Bojke *et al*. 2001) and all started operation as level 1 or level 2 PCGs.

The 3 years following 1999 saw many mergers between neighbouring PCGs and a very rapid process of transition to trust status, accelerated by the implementation of *Shifting the Balance of Power* (Department of Health 2001a). By the time of the fieldwork for the third Tracker Survey in early 2002, 66 per cent of the PCGs in the original sample had merged with neighbouring PCGs and 56 per cent of these had merged with two or more PCGs (Smith *et al*. 2002). The average population covered by PCG/Ts had doubled to approximately 200,000, with some PCG/Ts serving more than 300,000 people. Mergers were seen as a way of achieving both greater leverage or bargaining power and economies of scale. However, chief executives also recognized that there were associated costs, notably becoming more remote from key stakeholders (GPs, nurses and other primary care professionals), a loss of local focus and the challenges of managing organizational change. Mergers often coincided with the transition from PCG to PCT status. By the time of the third Tracker Survey, 45 per cent of the original PCG sample had become PCTs and the remainder made the change in April 2002. All had opted for level 4 trust status, enabling them to both provide and commission services (Smith *et al*. 2002). All had become providers of community nursing services and most were also providing a range of other community health services, including intermediate care (85 per cent), health promotion (77 per cent), chiropody (77 per cent) and physiotherapy (61 per cent).

In the space of only 3 years, these newly formed organizations therefore underwent a massive process of organizational change and development. Yet there was little evidence of these changes being informed by a process of developmental learning or by the demonstration of their capacity to take on new roles, both of which were advocated in the White Paper (Secretary of State for Health 1997). Much of the effort during their first year as PCGs was taken up with establishing the new organization and getting the PCG board to function effectively (Wilkin and Sheaff 1999). In many cases, mergers have doubled or even trebled the constituencies of local GPs, nurses and other health professionals, and have required the appointment of new boards and many associated committees and working groups (such as clinical governance, information management and technology, primary care development, prescribing, commissioning). At the same time, the transition from PCG to PCT status has required significant changes in governance arrangements, including the appointment of non-executive board members and members of the new professional executive committee. There have also been significant changes in the managerial leadership of PCTs. As well as the appointment of a lay chair of the new trust board, only 17 per cent of the PCG/Ts in the Tracker Survey retained the same chief executive or chair of the PCG board and PCT professional executive committee throughout the 3-year period from 1999 to 2002 (Smith *et al*. 2002).

The scale of organizational development was reflected in the staffing levels of PCG/Ts over the 3 years. In 1999, most PCGs were small organizations, some employing only one or two staff in addition to a chief executive.

More than half (53 per cent) of the PCGs in the Tracker Survey sample employed less than five staff in the 1999/2000 financial year and only 9 per cent employed more than eight staff. However, by the time of the third Tracker Survey, only two PCGs employed less than five staff and the average number of core managerial, finance and administrative staff employed had risen to 11.3 in PCGs and 31.5 in PCTs. In addition, PCTs assumed responsibility for large numbers of clinical and administrative staff providing community health services. The average number of such staff in PCTs was 269, with a range of 98 to 562 (Smith *et al.* 2002). Of course, as well as supporting increased capacity, this rapid growth in the size and complexity of the new primary care organizations generated its own additional demands, with the need to develop appropriate management structures, human resource management, internal communication and information management systems (see Chapter 8), and to clarify roles and responsibilities in relation to these internal functions.

Despite the rapid growth in the number and range of staff employed by PCG/Ts, 61 per cent of chief executives questioned in the third Tracker Survey reported that their current staffing levels were inadequate. Indeed, the lack of organizational capacity, particularly shortages of staff, topped the list of obstacles and barriers to progress given by chief executives in each of the three surveys; the number mentioning this increased from 40 per cent of PCGs in the first year to 61 per cent in the third year. The most common aspect of this inadequate organizational infrastructure was a lack of management capacity, although all chief executives cited some combination of shortage of staff, constraints on overall resources, the pace of change and the amount and complexity of organizational change. There appeared to be a widening gap between the expectations on PCGs and PCTs to deliver organizational change, better services and improved health and their capacity to do so (Dowling *et al.* 2002).

Central control versus local autonomy

The government's intention in creating PCGs and PCTs was to place GPs, nurses and local communities at the forefront of developing and providing local health services, using the unified budget to deploy resources flexibly to strengthen local services and ensure that patterns of care best reflect patients' needs (Secretary of State for Health 1997; NHS Executive 1998). The publication in 2001 of *Shifting the Balance of Power in the NHS* (Department of Health 2001a) restated the government's claim to be devolving power to frontline staff and local communities 'so that they reconnect with their services and have real influence over their development' (p. 5).

At the same time, the government sought to address a perceived breakdown in national standards believed to have been a consequence of the market reforms of the 1990s, resulting in so-called 'postcode inequities' between patients in different health authorities and a 'two-tier' service for the patients of fundholding and non-fundholding practices. Thus *Shifting the Balance of Power in the NHS* (Department of Health 2001a) asserted that frontline staff needed to be in charge of frontline services and have the managerial power to meet local communities' needs – always within the context of clear national standards and a strong accountability framework. The rapid development of PCTs between 1999 and 2002 has, therefore, been accompanied by the emergence of increasingly prescriptive national standards, targets and guidelines. The *NHS Plan* (Secretary of State for Health 2000), national service frameworks (Department of Health 1999, 2000, 2001b, c), guidelines on treatment issued by the National Institute for Clinical Excellence, the inspection regime undertaken by the Commission for Health Improvement, and the NHS performance management system for trusts, all place requirements on PCTs to conform to centrally prescribed policies and priorities.

One of the initial attractions of PCGs and PCTs to health professionals was the prospect of replacing the centralized and hierarchical governance structures that had characterized the NHS more or less since its foundation with a more open and participatory model of governance that would permit greater local autonomy. Although the NHS internal market of the 1990s allowed limited freedom to fundholding practices, it should be remembered that four-fifths of the budget for hospital services remained with the health authorities, as did the budget for GP services. In the first Tracker Survey of PCGs covering 1999/2000, those planning to become PCTs were asked their reasons for making the transition. Just over half (52 per cent) cited achieving independence from their local health authority and a further 27 per cent said that they saw PCT status as an opportunity to focus their attention on local needs and services (Wilkin and Coleman 1999). By the second year of the Tracker Survey, 49 per cent of PCGs cited focusing on local needs and services as a reason for wanting to move to trust status (Coleman and Wilkin 2001).

However, the opportunities for either PCGs or PCTs to focus on local health needs and priorities for service development have been constrained by an increasingly prescriptive national policy agenda. In the third round of the Tracker Survey, for which the fieldwork was conducted between January and March 2002, chairs of PCG boards and PCT professional executive committees were asked to assess the relative influence of national and local priorities. Over two-thirds (69 per cent) rated national policies, priorities and targets as having the strongest influence, while only 5 per cent said that local priorities were more influential. The majority (90 per cent) wanted greater opportunities to focus on local health needs and service development priorities. Examples of local priorities included rural deprivation and transport problems, mental health services, deprived populations and the needs of ethnic minority patients (Smith *et al*. 2002). Although the perceived support of GPs and nurses for their local PCG/T remained quite strong in 2002 (Smith *et al*. 2002), it is questionable whether this will continue to be the case if the dominance of national targets over local priorities persists in the longer term. Local issues are likely to affect the work of GPs and nurses on an almost daily basis, and the importance of national targets may appear less relevant to them.

Managing the financial framework

The creation of PCG/Ts was associated with major changes in the budgetary framework of the NHS. Previously, budgets for hospital services, prescribing and GP services were separated and held by a mixture of health authorities and fundholding practices. Expenditure on general medical services was determined by a combination of the number of GPs, demand from patients and the behaviour of GPs (for example, in the use of laboratory tests and X-rays). The budgets of PCTs are moving towards a more equitable capitation formula, in which all elements of the budget will reflect local health needs and levels of deprivation. A potentially even more significant change is the allocation of a unified budget to PCTs, to replace the former separate budgets for prescribing, hospital and community health services, and general practice infrastructure. The total pot of money generated for each PCT by the new resource allocation formulae can, therefore, now be spent on any of the previously separate budget headings in proportions decided by the PCT, rather than the available amounts for specific functions being determined – and limited – by the size of that particular budget. This reform of the budgetary framework is an essential element of the policy to shift decision-making to more local levels, as it gives PCTs greater flexibility in deciding how money should be spent in the provision of local services.

Primary care trusts, and the PCGs before them, therefore have two key tasks: to decide whether to use the new financial flexibilities to transfer funds between the former separate budget headings of hospital and community health services, general practice infrastructure and prescribing; and to establish systems for controlling expenditure, providing incentives to practices and managing risks (Dusheiko *et al.* 2002). The third round of the Tracker Survey addressed these issues by examining PCG/Ts' strategic management of their unified budgets through the shifting of expenditure; the development of methods for managing financial risk; and their use of incentive schemes to promote change.

As implied earlier, the freedom to shift expenditure between hospital and community health services, prescribing and general practice infrastructure is a fundamental aspect of devolved financial decision-making in the 'new' NHS. Some PCG/Ts had already made changes in the pattern of expenditure between different budget heads by 2002, and most were planning to make changes in the future. The main trend in planned changes to expenditure was to increase spending on primary and community services (Figure 6.3). In some cases, this could be achieved through the allocation of new funding, but 40 per

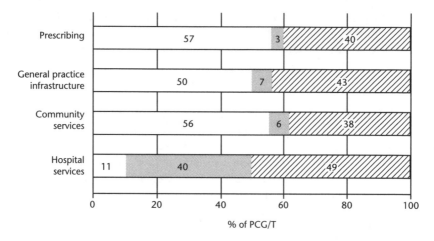

Figure 6.3 Percentages of PCG/Ts planning shifts in expenditure. ❑, planning increase; ❑, planning decrease; ❑, no change planned.

cent of PCG/Ts were planning to reduce spending on hospital provision. Because GPs have a central role in the governance of PCG/Ts, it is perhaps not surprising that resources are being shifted towards primary and community health services, since these are the main concerns of GPs (Dusheiko *et al.* 2002). In general, though, these plans to change expenditure from inherited patterns suggest that the new primary care organizations were beginning to think strategically about their management of the unified budget.

The smaller the population covered, the more demand for health services is prone to fluctuations. Even with populations of around 200,000, PCTs are still not immune from fluctuating demand, making it necessary for them to adopt strategies for managing the potential financial consequences. One mechanism for managing such risk is to be able to carry forward overspends and underspends from year to year. Yet nearly half (48 per cent) of PCG/Ts in 2001/2 were not allowed by their health authorities to carry forward over-spends or underspends. A third (34 per cent) were allowed to carry forward underspends only, just 12 per cent could carry forward overspends only, and only 5 per cent were able to carry forward both overspends and underspends. These restrictions on the ability to manage fluctuations in expenditure may become a serious obstacle to financial management in smaller PCTs (Dusheiko *et al.* 2002).

With primary care organizations expected to take on responsibility for some three-quarters of the NHS budget, the use of financial incentives to shape the expenditure-related behaviour of general practices and providers of secondary care services is likely to become an important tool for managing budgets. Prescribing is the second largest item of expenditure after hospital and community health services, and all PCTs are required to operate a prescribing incentive scheme designed to reward effective and efficient prescribing by GPs. In 2001/2, 83 per cent of PCG/Ts had established rewards for practices that were linked to both financial and quality prescribing targets. Primary care trusts also have opportunities to control expenditure by offering incentives to their constituent general practices to curb spending on hospital and community health services costs by, for example, controlling referrals. Progress here has been slow, with only one in ten PCG/Ts having introduced such incentives by 2001/2 and 59 per cent having no plans to introduce them. Moreover, most PCG/Ts (88 per cent) had also not introduced any financial incentives into service agreements with providers through the commissioning process by 2001/2 (see Chapter 9). However, 48 per cent of PCG/Ts reported that they had included financial incentives to improve services into personal medical services contracts and 65 per cent reported already using financial incentives to improve the quality of services through their clinical governance framework (see Chapter 7). Overall, the evidence on the reported use of financial incentives is mixed, with incentives being common in some areas of activity but rare in others (Dusheiko et al. 2002).

These various mechanisms for PCTs to manage their budgets need to be located within the context of the overarching mechanisms for financial allocation and the control of expenditure. Leaving aside possible disagreements about the level at which the unified budgets have been set, a comparison between expenditure and budgets is the most common measure for good financial management. Just under half (46 per cent) of PCG/Ts reported that their expenditure for the financial year 2000/1 was more or less in line with their budget allocation for the year (Dusheiko et al. 2002), with 33 per cent reporting underspends and 21 per cent overspends. Movement towards target budget levels, based on health needs and levels of deprivation as reflected in weighted capitation formulae, is proceeding slowly. Budgets for many PCG/Ts in the first 3 years reflected historical spending patterns, rather than the target levels determined by weighted capitation. However, by early 2002, 37 per cent of PCG/T chief executives expected their expenditure for the financial year 2001/2 to be more or less the same as their target allocation. A further 46 per cent expected expenditure to be within 5 per cent of the target allocation (33 per cent above target and 13 per cent below target). Only 22 per cent expected expenditure to be more than 5 per cent outside the target (17 per cent over target and 5 per cent below target).

An important factor determining the effectiveness of PCG/Ts in managing their budgets is the number of staff employed in their finance departments. The number of finance staff employed by PCG/Ts steadily increased over their first 3 years. In 2000/1, 15 per cent of PCG/Ts had no directly employed finance staff and employed an average of only one whole time equivalent.

By 2002, only 9 per cent (all PCGs) had no finance staff and the average complement had risen to three whole time equivalents. Seventy-three per cent of PCG/Ts also employed directors of finance. As would be expected, variations between PCG/Ts in the numbers of finance staff they employed could be partly explained by differences in the size of the populations they covered and hence their total budgets (Smith *et al.* 2002). However, despite the increases in finance staff, 61 per cent of PCG/T chief executives still claimed in 2002 that their overall staffing levels were inadequate and 48 per cent said they would give high priority to employing more finance staff.

Conclusions

Primary care trusts are an important experiment in devising an alternative system of organizing and governing health care in the NHS, an experiment that will also offer lessons to other countries outside England (see Chapter 3). Primary care has a central role in driving the modernization agenda for the NHS as a whole, so strong organizations that reflect and represent the different interests within the sector will be required to achieve the ambitious targets relevant to the government's reforms.

Progress has been made in building management capacity in primary care organizations since 1999, although this has been accompanied by a growth both in the targets they need to achieve and in the range of their responsibilities. However, as many PCG/T chief executives considered their organizations still to be understaffed in 2002, it is possible their workload since 1999 may have increased faster than their staffing and other aspects of organizational capacity. The large numbers of mergers, and the faster than expected transition from PCG to PCT status, have also placed tremendous strains on relatively new organizations. In relation to the management of their budgets, PCG/Ts do appear to be controlling spending effectively, as shown in the narrowed gap between target resource allocations and actual expenditure. There is also evidence of development in strategic thinking about the unified budget that PCTs now formally control.

As might be expected, there is evidence of variation in the influence of different groups of stakeholders in PCG/Ts. While the continuing relatively high levels of support for PCG/Ts among the various professional stakeholders implies an absence of any serious tensions between GPs and nurses, the prospect of such problems arising in the future should not be ignored. Problems may also arise in sustaining the continued support of GPs, who, as PCGs became PCTs, appeared to lose some influence relative to managers. Difficulties in sustaining the support of frontline professional stakeholders may have been increased by the widespread mergers between PCG/Ts; by 2001/2, the average population of PCTs was approximately double that of PCGs in 1999.

Large organizations can appear more remote to local stakeholders than smaller bodies, although locality groups are being established to alleviate some of these problems. Nonetheless, to keep local stakeholders 'on board', it is likely that PCTs will need to work hard at establishing a new identity that is distinctively different from that of the old health authorities.

Furthermore, PCTs will also need to avoid recreating at local levels the old command and control structure of the NHS that has continued to characterize the service to a greater or lesser extent, even during the market reforms of the 1990s. Retaining the participation of local stakeholders in the new organizational structures of primary care may also be threatened by the greater priority given to national policy over local concerns within the organizational and developmental agendas of PCTs. This is liable to create tensions, as centrally set targets may not always be perceived as relevant by frontline staff and could thus result in a loss of interest in the reforms by local stakeholders. Indeed, this problem may also reflect wider features of the current 'modernization' agenda. There may be a fundamental tension between the aim of shifting the balance of power to frontline staff and the expectation that primary care organizations will willingly prioritize national targets over local priorities. Ultimately, frontline staff may find their newly devolved powers are simply the power to implement government policy, rather than developing locally decided strategies.

References

Bojke, C., Gravelle, H. and Wilkin, D. (2001) Is bigger better for primary care groups and trusts?, *British Medical Journal*, 322(7286): 599–602.

Coleman, A. and Wilkin, D. (2001) Organizational change: PCG mergers and progress to trust status, in D. Wilkin, S. Gillam and A. Coleman (eds) *The National Tracker Survey of Primary Care Groups and Trusts 2000/2001: Modernising the NHS*. Manchester: The University of Manchester.

Department of Health (1998) *A First Class Service: Quality in the New NHS*. London: Department of Health.

Department of Health (1999) *National Service Framework for Mental Health: Modern Standards and Service Models*. London: Department of Health.

Department of Health (2000) *National Service Framework for Coronary Heart Disease: Modern Standards and Service Models*. London: Department of Health.

Department of Health (2001a) *Shifting the Balance of Power in the NHS: Securing Delivery*. London: Department of Health.

Department of Health (2001b) *National Service Framework for Older People: Modern Standards and Service Models*. London: Department of Health.

Department of Health (2001c) *National Service Framework for Diabetes: Standards, Modern Standards and Service Models*. London: Department of Health.

Dowling, B., Wilkin, D. and Coleman, A. (2002) Management in primary care groups and trusts, *British Journal of Health Care Management*, 8(1): 12–5.

Dusheiko, M., Gravelle, H., Jacobs, R., Smith, P. and Dowling, B. (2002) Budgets and incentives, in D. Wilkin, A. Coleman, B. Dowling and K. Smith (eds) *The National Tracker Survey of Primary Care Groups and Trusts 2001/2002: Taking Responsibility?* Manchester: The University of Manchester.

Ham, C. (1992) *Health Policy in Britain: The Politics and Organisation of the National Health Service*. London: Macmillan.

NHS Executive (1998) The New NHS Modern and Dependable: Developing Primary Care Groups, *Health Service Circular HSC 1998/139*. Leeds: NHSE.

NHS Executive (1999) *Primary Care Trusts: Establishment, the Preparatory Period and their Functions*. London: Department of Health.

Secretary of State for Health (1997) *The New NHS: Modern, Dependable*. London: The Stationery Office.

Secretary of State for Health (2000) *The NHS Plan: A Plan for Investment, A Plan for Reform*. London: The Stationery Office.

Smith, K., Coleman, A., Dowling, B. and Wilkin, D. (2002) Organizational development and governance, in D. Wilkin, A. Coleman, B. Dowling and K. Smith (eds) *The National Tracker Survey of Primary Care Groups and Trusts 2001/2002: Taking Responsibility?* Manchester: The University of Manchester.

Wilkin, D. and Coleman, A. (1999) Trusts and mergers, in D. Wilkin, S. Gillam and B. Leese (eds) *The National Tracker Survey of Primary Care Groups and Trusts: Progress and Challenges 1999/2000*. Manchester: The University of Manchester.

Wilkin, D. and Sheaff, R. (1999) Organizational development and governance, in D. Wilkin, S. Gillam and B. Leese (eds) *The National Tracker Survey of Primary Care Groups and Trusts: Progress and Challenges 1999/2000*. Manchester: The University of Manchester.

Wilkin, D., Coleman, A., Dowling, B. and Smith, K. (eds) (2002) *The National Tracker Survey of Primary Care Groups and Trusts 2001/2002: Taking Responsibility?* Manchester: The University of Manchester.

7 Improving the quality of health care through clinical governance

Stephen Campbell and Martin Roland

Introduction: why improve quality of care?

Improving the quality of care is important to maximize health in the population; to enhance efficiency (ineffective care wastes resources); to minimize errors (which cause unnecessary morbidity and mortality); to maximize the effectiveness of care (to produce desired health outcomes) and to ensure accountability (of health professionals and managers). There is evidence of significant variation in the quality of primary health care (Seddon *et al.* 2001), of medical errors (Alberti 2001) and examples of unacceptable standards of primary care (Bahrami and Evans 2001; Josebury *et al.* 2001). In addition, the rise of consumerism (with a concomitant reduction in professional power) acts as a catalyst for change, as does the current value of negligence claims against the National Health Service (NHS), which stands at £2.5 billion. Pressures to improve the quality of health care are further fuelled by the public unease resulting from media coverage of high-profile cases in the NHS, such as the Shipman murder trial and the Bristol Inquiry into the high mortality rates of childhood heart surgery (Smith 1998). In essence, there are systematic problems with the quality of a service that was previously taken largely for granted. The modernization agenda of the government includes a strong commitment to improving the quality of health care through the mechanism of clinical governance.

In this chapter, we discuss the concept of clinical governance, how it has been implemented by primary care groups and trusts (PCG/Ts) to date and the prospects for its success in improving the quality of health care.

Clinical governance

Clinical governance is part of a 10-year strategy for improving the quality of care provided by the NHS, which began in 1997. It is a cornerstone of

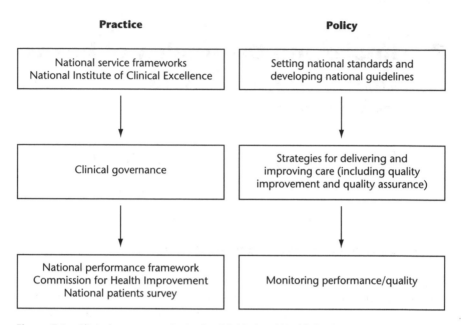

Figure 7.1   Clinical governance in the English National Health Service.

the Labour government's modernization programme for the NHS, affecting all health organizations and all health professionals. Clinical governance is defined as 'a framework through which NHS organizations are accountable for continually improving the quality of their services, safeguarding high standards by creating an environment in which excellence in clinical care will flourish' (Department of Health 1998: 33). This framework includes both assessing and monitoring existing care to ensure minimum standards are being met and improving future care (Secretary of State for Health 2000). It involves three distinct but overlapping elements (Figure 7.1).

The first element of this quality framework is the development of national standards and guidelines to foster improvements in, and standardize, care. The framework is developed through two key mechanisms, the national service frameworks and the National Institute for Clinical Excellence (NICE).

National service frameworks are service level (relating to the whole of the NHS in England) models, which set minimum standards for the delivery and monitoring of health services, including primary care. They confer a statutory duty on all NHS organizations. By the end of 2002, several national service frameworks had been published, including those for mental health (Department of Health 1999a), coronary heart disease (Department of Health 2000a) and diabetes (Department of Health 2002a).

The National Institute for Clinical Excellence was established in 1999 to undertake and publish evidence-based appraisals of clinical interventions and clinical guidelines for medical conditions such as diabetes, coronary heart disease, asthma and depression (Hutchinson *et al.* 2000). It has also published over forty technology appraisals, mostly relating to the use of medicines. Since January 2002 PCG/Ts, which now have responsibility for managing the quality and costs of prescribing, have had a statutory obligation to fund treatments recommended by NICE.

The second component of the quality framework involves approaches that seek to improve care and prevent poor care on a continuous basis as part of everyday routine practice. The process of clinical governance embraces many previous approaches, including, audit; learning from complaints by patients or adverse events (where something has gone wrong); performance indicators; clinical guidelines; patient surveys; education and training; and continuous professional development. However, clinical governance seeks to universalize these previously often fragmented approaches (Scally and Donaldson 1998); and to combine previous professional approaches to measuring and improving quality of care (such as clinical audit) and managerial approaches (such as risk management) (Buetow and Roland 1999; Sheaff 2001) within a single, systems-based strategy. The approaches being used by PCG/Ts are discussed below.

The third part of the framework is concerned with monitoring the existing care provided by NHS organizations and practitioners, to ensure that it meets minimum standards – for example, that the targets stipulated in national service frameworks are being met. This includes identifying those whose performance does not meet these standards.

There are three main components of this monitoring framework. The national performance framework is a series of high-level performance indicators, originally designed to be applied at a health authority level for populations of between 200,000 and 500,000 (NHS Executive 1999). These have now been supplemented by PCG/T-level indicators (Department of Health 2002b) that evaluate progress in improving quality of care. In addition, the Commission for Health Improvement and Assessment (CHIA; originally named the Commission for Health Improvement) was set up in 1999 to conduct a rolling programme of reviews of NHS organizations, including hospitals and general practices. Trust reviews include the level of adherence to national service framework standards and compliance with NICE guidance. The Commission for Health Improvement and Assessment will also publish comparative information about NHS organizations and consistent poor performance may result in the imposition of sanctions, including the replacement of managerial and/ or clinical leaders. Finally, the government has committed itself to carrying out national patient surveys that would allow systematic comparisons of the experience of patients and their carers over time and between different parts of the country (Department of Health 1997). Although these surveys have not been conducted annually, one was conducted in 1998 that included primary care and national surveys have also been carried out relating to cancer care and coronary heart disease. A survey of patients' experiences of primary care was repeated in 2002.

Other elements of this regulatory framework include the proposed revalidation of doctors' professional registration and compulsory appraisal of general practitioners (GPs) (Salter 2001). In addition, the NHS has adopted a policy of controls assurance, which seeks to ensure that organizations are well managed in both financial and clinical terms (Department of Health 1999b). Lastly, since April 2002, 28 new strategic health authorities are responsible for managing the performance of PCG/Ts in their area.

The accountability of PCG/Ts for clinical governance therefore formally extends 'upwards' (for example, the performance of PCG/Ts managed by strategic health authorities), 'downwards' (for example, care provided to patients and local communities is assessed by national service frameworks and patient surveys) and also horizontally, to peers (for example, through peer assessments and shared learning and data).

Primary care groups and trusts are responsible for implementing clinical governance in primary and community health care, as well as in secondary (hospital-based) care. Although clinical governance affects all health professionals and organizations, this chapter focuses upon PCG/Ts and the implementation of clinical governance in primary care and, more specifically, general practice. This is because, despite the diverse workforce and responsibilities of PCG/Ts, they are the lead NHS organizations for assessing need, planning health services and improving primary and community health in their localities (Department of Health 1997).

The data presented in this chapter draw upon the longitudinal Tracker Survey. As described in Chapter 1, this followed a sample of PCG/Ts in England, with fieldwork in 1999/2000, 2000/1 and 2001/2. In each year of data collection, questionnaires were sent to the member of the PCG/T board with lead responsibility for clinical governance; response rates were 78 per cent, 81 per cent and 72 per cent respectively. Data are presented for the 2001/2 survey except where indicated, as well as findings from research undertaken elsewhere.

Clinical governance priorities

Guidance from NICE and the national service frameworks have significantly influenced the way clinical governance is being implemented by PCG/Ts. Strategies to improve and monitor adherence to such guidance and standards have been a core activity of many PCG/Ts. Clinical areas covered by the national service frameworks were the main targets for clinical governance priorities in 94 per cent of PCG/Ts in 2001/2. Reflecting the publication of successive national service frameworks, coronary heart disease has been the highest

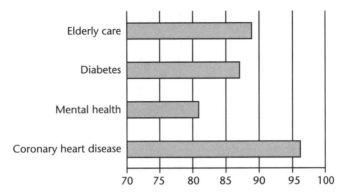

Figure 7.2 Percentages of PCG/Ts with strategies to implement national service frameworks in 2001/2.

clinical priority for PCG/Ts since 1999/2000, followed by mental health care, diabetes and elderly care, with the latter particularly increasing its profile since 2000/1.

The importance of the national service frameworks is reflected by the fact that most clinical governance leads report having developed or being in the process of developing protocols, guidelines and service agreements for their implementation (Figure 7.2), and identifying staff with lead responsibility for clinical governance in these areas (Figure 7.3). There is also someone with lead governance responsibility for improving cancer care in 82 per cent of PCG/Ts.

Local influences on clinical governance priorities include guidance from PCG/T clinical governance working groups (90 per cent of PCG/Ts), prescribing priorities (65 per cent), health improvement priorities (56 per cent) and the concerns of local GPs (47 per cent) and nurses (33 per cent).

Strategies to implement clinical governance

A plethora of approaches have been used to implement clinical governance at the PCG/T level (Campbell *et al.* 2001; Sweeney *et al.* 2002). The most common strategies identified from the three Tracker surveys are shown in Figure 7.4.

Other strategies include sharing comparative data relevant to all general practices; benchmarking PCG/T and practice-level data with data from other PCG/Ts or practices; and the setting and monitoring of standards. In addition, 90 per cent of PCG/Ts are using significant event reporting (which investigates cases where things have gone wrong), promoting organizational audit (63 per cent), feeding back audit results to practices (71 per cent) and GP appraisal (35 per cent). These varied strategies fall into five main mechanisms for change. These are education and training (especially shared

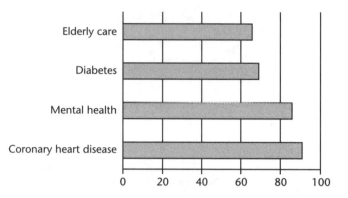

Figure 7.3 Percentages of PCG/Ts with individuals with lead responsibility for implementing clinical governance in areas covered by national service frameworks in 2002.

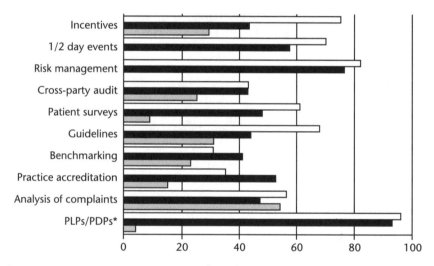

Figure 7.4 Percentages of PCG/Ts using different strategies to implement clinical governance.* (Personal learning plans/practice development plans.) ⬜, 2001/2; ◼, 2000/1; ⬜, 1999/2000.

learning), incentives, clinical guidelines, audit and the disclosure of practice level information.

Education and training

Most PCG/Ts are advocating strategies that seek to develop improvements in care through education, training and shared learning (Campbell *et al.* 2002; Sweeney *et al.* 2002). Regular half-day educational events, targeted either just at doctors or at all general practice staff, continue to be an important mechanism, increasing from 57 per cent of PCG/Ts in 2000/1 to 70 per cent in 2001/2. These initiatives promote shared learning between practices and reduce the isolation of practice staff. Attendance rates of over 95 per cent have been reported, even though participation is voluntary. Moreover, by 2001/2, over 90 per cent of PCG/Ts were providing education and training, as well as supporting the development of personal learning plans for GPs and nurses and practice development plans that focused on initiatives relevant to all staff in a general practice. Analysis of complaints by patients was also being encouraged by 57 per cent of PCG/Ts.

Other research has also found that PCG/Ts are deploying educational approaches for implementing clinical governance such as mentoring, and sharing experiences and learning (Sweeney *et al.* 2001, 2002). This is intended to nurture a sense of ownership, trust and voluntary engagement by practice staff. As one senior manager stated, 'We need to try to develop a rapport with all clinicians, to try and involve all professions and to try and develop an . . . atmosphere of trust' (Campbell *et al.* 2002: 10).

Incentive schemes

By 2001/2, 65 per cent of PCG/Ts were using – and a further 10 per cent were planning to use – incentive schemes relating to quality improvement (over and above prescribing incentive schemes). This figure compares with only 29 per cent in 1999/2000. The most common form of incentives are financial (89 per cent), with 26 per cent of PCG/Ts using non-financial incentives such as accreditation. Only 12 per cent of PCG/Ts were using both financial and non-financial incentives. While fewer than 10 per cent of financial incentive schemes offered less than £1000 per practice, 44 per cent provided £5000 or more, often weighted in terms of the numbers of patients registered with a practice. Among the 65 per cent of PCG/Ts that were using financial incentives in 2001/2, incentives were most commonly being used in relation to the targets set out in the national service frameworks for coronary heart disease (60 per cent), mental health (31 per cent) and elderly care (25 per cent), or for participating in audits (47 per cent). Other incentivized activities included attendance at PCG/T education or training events (37 per cent), formulating practice development plans (35 per cent) improved access to appointments (33 per cent) and, less frequently, patient evaluations of care (12 per cent).

Clinical guidelines and standards

Sixty-nine per cent of PCG/Ts were using clinical guidelines to be implemented across all the practices in their area in 2001/2. These corresponded to PCG/T clinical priorities for coronary heart disease (49 per cent of PCG/Ts), diabetes (22 per cent), mental health (10 per cent), statins/lipids (8 per cent), hypertension (8 per cent), asthma/chronic obstructive pulmonary disease (6 per cent) and cancer (6 per cent). Clinical guidelines were especially common in the local implementation of national service frameworks for coronary heart disease (65 per cent) and mental health (39 per cent).

Targets and standards were also being set by PCG/Ts in relation to non-clinical activities, such as waiting times for appointments with GPs (61 per cent) or other primary care staff (43 per cent), practice opening hours (31 per cent) and out-of-hours care (18 per cent).

Audit

Audit has been the most common quality improvement strategy used in England over the last 10 years. It is a systematic critical analysis of the quality of medical care, encompassing the procedures used for diagnosis and treatment, the use of resources and the resulting patient outcomes. Given this prominence, it is not surprising that cross-practice audit, where all practices within a PCG/T area take part, was being employed to see whether clinical guidelines were being met; 47 per cent of PCG/Ts in 2001/2 were offering practices financial incentives to undertake audits. However, PCG/Ts appear to be split on how to coordinate audit. For example, 46 per cent were stipulating to their practices that they should undertake audits in specified clinical areas, whereas 43 per cent were encouraging practices to undertake clinical audit but letting them choose the topic. Only 4 per cent of PCG/Ts were allowing practices to decide whether they wanted to conduct any clinical audit.

Information on quality of care

In 1999/2000, 47 per cent of PCG/Ts reported that they had plans to make data on quality of care publicly available. As Figure 7.5 shows, by 2000/1 many PCG/Ts were actively engaged in disclosing identifiable or anonymous information about the quality of care in their constituent general practices to the general public, other general practices and PCG/T boards. This mechanism reflects an increasing policy interest in the public disclosure of data generally (Marshall and Davies 2001). Although this strategy continued in 2001/2, it was more likely to involve the use of anonymous data rather than identifiable data. The more widespread use of anonymous as opposed to identifiable data suggests that clinical governance leads are perhaps tempering their initial plans for greater openness, after being faced with the practical issues this entails. There is, moreover, little evidence that the public release of comparative data improves quality of care in an English context (Marshall and Davies 2001). Indeed, it may be counterproductive if it creates a defensive culture among doctors (Davies and Lampel 1998) and could undermine the overall

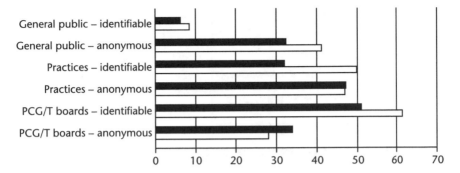

Figure 7.5 Percentages of PCG/Ts collecting anonymous and identifiable data on general practice performance. ■, 2001/2; ❑, 2000/1.

emphasis on supportive and developmental quality improvement strategies being advocated by PCG/Ts.

Although PCG/Ts may be retreating from publishing data in which individual practices are identifiable, this does not mean that PCG/Ts are not collecting data. Indeed, in 2001/2 PCG/Ts were collecting data from 'all or most practices' in their area in 96 per cent of cases for coronary heart disease, 83 per cent for diabetes, 75 per cent for access to/use of primary care, 53 per cent for hospital admissions, 43 per cent for mental health, 40 per cent for admissions, 23 per cent for cancer and 24 per cent for elderly care. Thirty-five per cent of PCG/Ts were offering their practices financial incentives to provide information on quality of care. Such data were used to compare the performance of all practices within a PCG/T as well as the performance of individual PCG/Ts with other PCG/Ts.

Systems for dealing with poor performance

In general, PCG/Ts appear to be promoting developmental, supportive and educational approaches to implementing clinical governance, backed up by mechanisms to monitor performance and quality, such as audit. This overall strategy extends to dealing with practices whose performance is perceived to be suboptimal, with PCG/Ts using informal discussions, training, clinical audit and offering extra resources for improvement (Figure 7.6). Identifying, managing and improving underperforming clinicians and practices are key policy aims of both the government (Department of Health 1999a, 2000b) and the Royal College of General Practitioners (2000).

However, by 2001/2, 20 per cent of PCG/Ts were advocating formal disciplinary procedures for dealing with poor care, compared with only 7 per cent in 2000/1. This confirms evidence from other research, where clinical

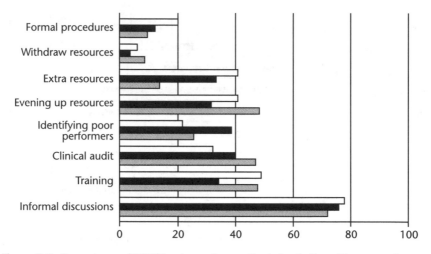

Figure 7.6 Percentages of PCG/Ts using various methods for dealing with poor performers. ❏, 2001/2; ■, 2000/1; ❏, 1999/2000.

governance leads admitted that formal procedures were being planned and were necessary, despite continuing to favour educational approaches (Campbell *et al.* 2002). In addition, all PCTs are required to have formal appraisal systems for GPs in place by 2003.

The increase in the use of formal procedures reflects the fact that chief executives of PCTs are legally responsible for the quality of care provided within their organization. Moreover, while many former PCGs left responsibility for formal procedures to health authorities, the latter have now been abolished. However, these formal procedures are, as yet, less well developed than quality improvement strategies (Campbell *et al.* 2002). One reason for this is that many clinical governance staff were initially unsure exactly what 'carrots or sticks' were at their disposal to monitor and improve the quality of care, to deal with incidences of substandard care or to encourage resistant colleagues to engage with clinical governance (Sweeney *et al.* 2002). Many PCG/T board members with lead responsibility for clinical governance initially lacked clarity about the levers available (for example, financial incentives or publication of league tables) and relied on the goodwill of their 'independent contractor' colleagues to move the process forward (Sweeney *et al.* 2002). Developmental approaches were, therefore, often the only possible option available to PCGs. However, the use of formal disciplinary procedures, financial incentives and public disclosure of data are now common mechanisms in PCG/Ts; the use of these levers has increased as the statutory responsibilities of PCG/Ts have grown. It is to be expected that they will be used more frequently in the future, in relation to both practices and individual practitioners, where supportive and educational approaches fail to improve the quality of care. The staff of

PCG/Ts are also aware that it is important to identify organizations where standards are not acceptable; as one lay board member of a PCG/T stated: 'At the end of the day, you have to demonstrate what you've done. And we're not just in the ministry of nice feelings . . . we need to see quality and excellence as a result' (Campbell *et al.* 2002: 11).

The prospects for the success of clinical governance

The roots of clinical governance can be seen in new public management initiatives begun in the 1980s (Hood 1995). These initiatives led to an increasing focus on the quality of public services, but this focus only became central to government policy in the late 1990s (Broadbent and Laughlin 1998; Kaboolian 1998). New public management enthusiasts argue that public sector services, including the NHS, should be subjected to managerial techniques imported from the private sector, such as contracts, cost containment, performance indicators and mechanisms to drive efficiency savings, as well as policy-making based on research evidence. This approach is not restricted to England but is an international phenomenon (Barberis 1998). However, clinical governance also constitutes some important departures from previous policies.

First, the framework is a mandatory requirement for all those who provide or manage patient care services in England. Previously, most approaches that had been used to measure and improve quality of care, such as audit, were voluntary (Buetow and Roland 1999; Sheaff 2001). However, the new clinical governance regime makes improving quality a duty of NHS organizations and their chief executives, which is equal to their other statutory responsibilities such as financial probity (Freeman 2002). Chief executives of PCG/Ts are now responsible for the clinical as well as the financial performance of their organizations.

Secondly, unlike previous quality initiatives that were undertaken at health authority, hospital, trust, general practice or individual practitioner level, clinical governance represents the first coherent, systems-based strategy covering the NHS as a whole and relevant to all health practitioners. In the past, primary and community services in the NHS have been fragmented, and general practices have not usually worked together as part of larger organizations.

Because it embraces many previous approaches for improving quality of care, such as audit, guidelines, patient surveys and continuous professional development, clinical governance has been referred to as a 'new label for old ingredients' (Smith and Harris 1999). However, the new strategic approach to clinical governance seeks to universalize and combine these previously often fragmented policies within a systems-based strategy (Scally and Donaldson 1998; Buetow and Roland 1999; Sheaff 2001). So far there is little evidence of improvements in primary care; little data has yet been collected from which it is possible to conclude whether clinical governance has led to improvements in patient health outcomes (Le Grand 2002). The question remains, therefore, as to whether it will improve quality of care. Half way through the government's 10-year strategy to improve quality of care, there are causes for both optimism and concern.

Causes for optimism

There have been no previous systems-based initiatives of the type articulated by clinical governance, backed up with substantial resources and national policy commitments. Considerable progress has been made in establishing the culture and infrastructure necessary to deliver quality services and turn the rhetoric of clinical governance into reality. The government is championing national initiatives (for example, national service frameworks) and PCG/Ts are pursuing educational strategies (for example, practice development plans and cross-practice audits). As a result, a more transparent quality improvement agenda is emerging.

There are additional challenges to implementing clinical governance within general practice, in contrast, for example, to a hospital, primarily because of the tradition of the (often fiercely) independent contractor status enjoyed by GPs. Before the establishment of PCG/Ts, GPs worked largely independently of each other and practised within a self-regulated environment. One of the challenges that have faced PCG/Ts in implementing clinical governance has been to develop a more corporate culture, in which quality improvement became a shared enterprise. The evidence presented in this chapter suggests that this shared learning environment is beginning to take shape. There has been substantial progress in areas such as sharing data, conducting cross-practice audits and providing opportunities for general practice staff to learn together at PCG/T-sponsored educational events. These are all indicative of a major cultural change for primary care. This is a sound approach to take because education and learning at the organizational level have, in the case of general practices, been demonstrated to be effective methods of improving quality of care (Davies and Nutley 2000). Primary care groups and trusts appear to be aware of the need to address the underlying changes in behaviour and culture, both organizational and behavioural, that are required to create successful change (Marshall *et al.* 2002).

Moreover, PCG/Ts are employing multiple approaches to implementing clinical governance including, for example, audit, incentives and education and training. There is evidence that multi-level strategies for change that combine continuing education, audit and research are most likely to lead to changes in behaviour and quality of care (Calman 1998; Ferlie and Shortell 2001).

Until recently, financial incentives were used only in relation to pre-scribing behaviour (for example, rewarding the use of generic drugs), immunization and vaccination rates (such as immunization against measles, mumps and rubella, or influenza vaccination) and take-up rates for prevent-ive procedures such as cervical cytology screening. There is now evidence that PCG/Ts are linking financial incentives to a wider range of activities, such as audit or meeting the targets contained within the national service frameworks. Offering financial incentives is a realistic mechanism for get-ting practices to participate in quality improvement activities and it has been found previously to impact positively on the behaviour of doctors in England (Gosden *et al.* 2001). Incentives are likely to become increasingly important in the provision of primary care. The new contract for general practitioners proposes radical changes to the way in which GPs will be paid and services will be provided. The contract will be focused on the practice, not the individual GP, and between 30 and 50 per cent of GPs' remuner-ation may be linked to a complex set of quality targets and financial incen-tives that relate to clinical care provision and patient assessments of that care.

Improving the quality of care requires multi-level approaches to change, including the individual (e.g. general practitioner), the group or team (e.g. primary health care team or general practice), the overall organization (e.g. primary care trust) and the larger system (e.g. NHS) in which these individuals and organizations are embedded (Berwick 1996; Ferlie and Shortell 2001; Mechanic 2002). Coronary heart disease is a good exemplar for assessing the impact of clinical governance. It is a leading cause of death in the UK and, perhaps not surprisingly therefore, the predominant priority for many PCG/Ts. It is important to focus resources on both patients with established coronary heart disease (myocardial infarction or angina; i.e. secondary prevention) and those at high risk but without established disease (i.e. primary prevention). This is the main advantage of the systems-based model of clinical governance (Figure 7.7).

Causes for concern

Five years after the introduction of clinical governance, the concept remains vague and nebulous, even anodyne (Harrison 2002), requiring interpretation if it is to be operationalized on the ground (Campbell and Sweeney 2002). Indeed, clinical governance reflects both definitions of the word 'malleable'. On the one hand, it is capable of 'being shaped or formed' into different strat-egies, as is the case at the PCG/T level where a variety of approaches are being undertaken. On the other hand, it is also easily 'controlled or influenced', for example by national policy initiatives, such as national service frameworks. This has created a number of tensions within the 'systems-based' framework

---

National level

  • National Service Framework (influence on CG priorities in 94% of PCG/Ts)
  • NICE guidelines (influence on CG priorities in 65% of PCG/Ts)
  • Monitored by CHIA

PCG/T level

  • Protocol for the systematic assessment, treatment and follow-up of people with CHD (96% of PCG/Ts)
  • Financial incentives to take part in quality improvement (60%)
  • Collecting information from *all or most practices* in 96% of PCG/Ts
  • Local education and training events (53%)
  • Promoting organizational audit (35%).

Practice level

  • Practice clinical governance leads in all or most practices in 92% of PCG/Ts
  • Registers in all or most practices in 96% of PCG/Ts

(Data from 2001/2 Tracker Survey)

Figure 7.7   Implementing clinical governance for coronary heart disease (CHD) in a systems-based model. CG = clinical governance.

described above, which have potentially deleterious consequences for the successful implementation of clinical governance.

First, the imprecise nature of clinical governance potentially offers the kind of flexibilities that encourage local adaptation and ownership, foster organic growth and enable the development of individualized, boundary-crossing strategies appropriate for bringing about quality improvement in different localities. Primary care groups and trusts are, indeed, involved in a variety of these locally tailored initiatives. However, the government's policies for the NHS have been criticized for involving increased specification, stand-ardization and centralization of control (Harrison 2002; Le Grand 2002). Evidence from the Tracker surveys suggests that PCG/Ts may be focusing upon national service framework priority areas at the expense of local priorities (Banks-Smith *et al.* 2002). Moreover, research using a purposive sample of 12 PCG/Ts (Campbell *et al.* 2002) has shown that, while in theory PCG/Ts have discretion over how they implement clinical governance, some senior managers are sceptical about how much flexibility they have in practice. As one PCG board member with lead responsibility for clinical governance stated, 'I think the government's approach is . . . all about performance management. The trouble with that, which is very much a top-down approach, is that if you're not careful you can squash out all the innovations' (p. 12). Other managers in this study emphasized that they had had to focus on government-set targets, such as reducing waiting lists for cancer patients which, while important, were nationally-set priorities at the expense of local priorities. The government's centralizing approach is, therefore, at odds with the predominately educational and local approaches to quality improvement being advocated by PCG/Ts.

Second, while research has shown that PCG/Ts have endeavoured to establish a no-blame, supportive culture (Sweeney *et al.* 2002), they have also been putting in place the infrastructure for monitoring service provision (Campbell *et al.* 2002). This is because performance management is 'front and centre' of the government's reform plans for the NHS (Smith 2002). However, there is a risk that such a heavy hand of control will inhibit positive change (Le Grand 2002). Indeed, there is evidence that some PCG/Ts have had difficulties reconciling their dual roles of supporting and monitoring the care provided by their constituent organizations and practitioners (Campbell *et al.* 2002). This is aggravated by the fact that strategies to improve care in England have usually been associated by health professionals with performance management (Freeman 2002). Professionals may be unwilling to participate in quality improvement strategies if they perceive them to be a means of blaming other professionals for things that go wrong (Shekelle 2002). This tension is illustrated in Figure 7.8. In future, PCTs will need to get the balance right between enabling practitioners and organizations to improve the quality of care within a supportive, no-blame environment, while simultaneously monitoring care to ensure that it does not fall below minimum standards.

Third, there are several other issues and barriers that threaten to undermine the success of clinical governance; these need addressing if it is to maximize its potential (Figure 7.9). In particular, the successful implementation of clinical governance will require sustainable and robust infrastructures, backed up by adequate resources, both human and financial. However, 42 per cent of PCG/Ts had no dedicated budget for clinical governance in 2001/2. Where they did exist, budgets ranged from £13,000 to £400,000, with a mean of £96,826 (£23,000 in 2000, £15,000 in 1999). (The increase in the mean budget is perhaps a reflection of the higher number of PCTs in the Tracker sample in 2002 (54 per cent) than in 2000 (8 per cent).) It was thus not surprising that four-fifths of respondents to the 2001/2 Tracker survey mentioned shortage of resources as the biggest obstacle to the successful implementation of clinical governance: 'lack of resources, funds and human time'; 'inadequate resources – lack of administrative and support staff'; or simply 'time, money'.

The perceived constraint of resources was compounded by the perception of an ever-growing agenda: 'number of must-do's are overwhelming practices', 'massive agenda – constantly struggling to prioritize'. These pressures reflect the fact that the implementation of clinical governance by PCG/Ts has been undertaken within an environment of continuing organizational change, as

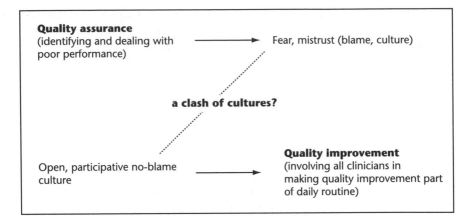

Figure 7.8   Reconciling quality assurance and quality improvement.

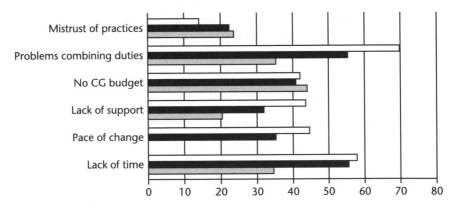

Figure 7.9   Percentages of PCG/Ts reporting barriers to implementing clinical governance. CG = clinical governance. ❑, 2001/2; ■, 2000/1; ❑, 1999/2000.

the implementation of the national service frameworks continues and pro-posals are developed for the revalidation of GPs. The pace of change was seen as a significant barrier by 45 per cent of clinical governance leads. The implementation of clinical governance in PCG/Ts, a major policy and organizational change in itself, has not occurred in a national policy vacuum, and PCG/Ts have not had the opportunity to consolidate their achievements, thereby risking the disengagement of both PCG/T and general practice staff. Many clinical governance leads reported that they did not have enough time to achieve all they had to do (an increase from 36 per cent in 1999/2000 to 57 per cent in 2001/2).

By early 2002, 71 per cent of PCG/Ts had one clinical governance lead and 29 per cent had two or more clinical governance leads. Of these leads, 81 per cent were GPs and 14 per cent were nurses. Most leads spent 3–5 hours (25 per cent) or 6–10 hours (40 per cent) a week on their role, but 15 and 19 per cent spent 11–15 hours or more than 15 hours per week, respectively. Moreover, there are signs of overload in the system, with many leads feeling unsupported in their role. Seventy per cent reported in 2001/2 that they found it difficult to combine their PCG/T commitments with their other commitments (an increase from 55 per cent in 2000/1 and from 36 per cent in 1999/2000). Moreover, 20 per cent and 22 per cent respectively reported in 2001/2 that they lacked the administrative or professional support necessary to implement clinical governance (the same as in 2000/1). Only per 6 per cent of clinical governance leads felt that they had a lot of support.

Other research has also shown that clinical governance leads feel unsupported. Wilson and Neary (2002) conducted a workshop with over 40 leads and found that many thought that there was not enough time to implement clinical governance and often inadequate support for clinical governance staff. Sweeney and colleagues (2002) have emphasized that clinical governance leads feel 'beleaguered' and are faced with a lack of funding, direction or guidance; a steep learning curve; long working hours; and a lack of time to absorb and understand multiple initiatives. These pressures have had an adverse impact on them personally, in terms of relationships both at home and at work.

There is also some evidence that PCG/Ts are finding it easier to implement some aspects of clinical governance (such as the standards within the national service framework for coronary heart disease) than others (for example, the standards within the national service framework for mental health) (Rogers *et al.* 2002). This may reflect the well-developed infrastructure for managing coronary heart disease within primary care compared to that for mental health, where mechanisms such as disease registers and audits are far less common.

The use of educational and supportive strategies by PCG/Ts appears to being paying some dividends. Mistrust by core practice staff (GPs, practice nurses, practice managers), a reported barrier to the successful implementation of clinical governance, has decreased from 25 per cent in 1999/2000 to 14 per cent in 2001/2, according to PCG/T clinical governance leads. More practices are actively engaged in clinical governance initiatives, working together and attending education and training events (Campbell *et al.* 2002; Marshall *et al.* 2002). They are also participating in cross-practice audits, especially for coronary heart disease, and there is a greater acceptance by many practice staff that routine data gathering is relevant to quality improvement. More practice staff have also become 'very supportive' or 'supportive' of clinical governance (at least according to clinical governance leads) since 1999 (Figure 7.10).

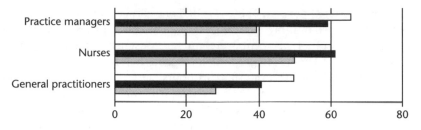

Figure 7.10 Percentages of core general practice staff 'very supportive' or 'supportive' of clinical governance. ❑, 2001/2; ■, 2000/1; ❑, 1999/2000.

However, one in seven clinical governance leads still feel that continued mistrust from practice staff acts as a barrier and that a significant minority of staff are still not supportive of clinical governance activities (Figure 7.10). Disengagement by health professionals from quality improvement activities is not limited to primary care but is endemic in health care – and not just in England (Shekelle 2002). This reinforces the arguments in favour of incremental and developmental approaches, underpinned by strategies that seek to create fundamental changes in organizational and behavioural (professional) cultures. However, these do not happen overnight – they take time to achieve (Davies *et al.* 2000), as does the creation of the necessary supporting systems and infrastructures to underpin them. Although there has been considerable progress in developing collective responsibility for improving quality of care – as manifest, for example, in shared learning activities – the independent contractor status of GPs and the fact that every practice has its own way of working may also undermine collective strategies (Marshall *et al.* 2002).

There is also some evidence that the infrastructure (the organizational factors that underpin the health system, such as finance, facilities and manpower) necessary to implement clinical governance in primary care is not in place. The need to improve the overall infrastructure of general practices has been highlighted by an Audit Commission report, which found significant variation in the quality of services accessed by patients. One in ten practices did not meet minimum standards and inner-city practices had poorer facilities and fewer doctors (Audit Commission 2002). The prevalence of organizational audit within PCG/T strategies for clinical governance suggests that clinical governance leads are addressing at least some of these variations in standards.

The government has acknowledged that clinical governance cannot be implemented overnight (Department of Health 1999b). Real improvements will accrue when resources and effort are accompanied by the organizational and cultural changes that are needed to improve quality of care. Three overlapping sets of issues need to be addressed simultaneously (Campbell and Sweeney 2002). First, the national context under which clinical governance is being implemented (the environment of change) must be clear, well resourced and allocated realistic timetables. Secondly, there must be leaders of clinical governance at the PCG/T level who are well supported, trained, enthusiastic and aware of the levers available to them. Thirdly, all health practitioners and managers will need to make clinical governance part of their daily routine. Not all health care staff can be (or need to be) leaders of clinical governance, but all staff must be users of the findings of clinical governance to ensure that all patients are beneficiaries of the framework.

Because clinical governance is not a single phenomenon but a constellation of local and national initiatives, it is difficult to judge its likely success or failure. Some strategies will fail and others will work. However, because clinical governance is a systems-based model, it is likely to be judged as a single entity, which will mask examples of both failure and success (Campbell and Sweeney 2002).

References

Alberti, K.G. (2001) Medical errors: a common problem. Is it time to get serious about them?, *British Medical Journal*, 322(7285): 501–2.

Audit Commission (2002) *A Focus on General Practice in England*. London: Audit Commission.

Bahrami, J. and Evans, A. (2001) Under performing doctors in general practice: a survey of referrals to UK Deaneries, *British Journal of General Practice*, 51(11): 892–6.

Banks-Smith, J., Shipman, C. and Gillam, S. (2002) What influence have national service frameworks had on the priorities of primary care groups and trusts?, *Journal of Clinical Governance*, 10(1): 7–11.

Barberis, P. (1998) The new public management and a new accountability, *Public Administration*, 76(3): 451–70.

Berwick, D.M. (1996) A primer on leading the improvement of systems, *British Medical Journal*, 312(7031): 619–22.

Broadbent, J. and Laughlin, R. (1998) Evaluating the 'New Public Management' reforms in the UK: a constitutional possibility?, *Public Administration*, 75(3): 487–507.

Buetow, S.A. and Roland, M.O. (1999) Clinical governance: bridging the gap between managerial and clinical approaches to quality of care, *Quality in Health Care*, 8(3): 184–90.

Calman, K. (1998) *A Review of Continuing Professional Development in General Practice: A Report by the Chief Medical Officer*. London: Department of Health.

Campbell, S.M. and Sweeney, G.M. (2002) The role of clinical governance as a strategy for quality improvement in primary care, *British Journal of General Practice*, 52 (suppl.): S12–S18.

Campbell, S.M., Roland, M.O. and Wilkin, D. (2001) Improving the quality of care through clinical governance, *British Medical Journal*, 322(7302): 1580–2.

Campbell, S.M., Sheaff, R., Sibbald, B. *et al.* (2002) Implementing clinical governance in English Primary Care Groups/Trusts: reconciling quality improvement and quality assurance, *Quality and Safety in Health Care*, 11(1): 9–14.

Davies, H.T.O. and Lampel, J. (1998) Trust in performance indicators?, *Quality in Health Care*, 7(3): 159–62.

Davies, H.T.O. and Nutley, S.M. (2000) Developing learning organisations in the new NHS, *British Medical Journal*, 320(7240): 998–1001.

Davies, H.T.O., Nutley, S.M. and Mannion, R. (2000) Organisational culture and quality of health care, *Quality in Health Care*, 9(2): 111–9.

Department of Health (1997) *A First Class Service: Quality in the new NHS*. London: Department of Health.

Department of Health (1999a) *National Service Framework for Mental Health: Modern Standards and Service Models*. London: Department of Health (http://www.doh.gov.uk/nsf).

Department of Health (1999b) *Clinical Governance: Quality in the New NHS*. London: Department of Health.

Department of Health (1999c) *Supporting Doctors, Protecting Patients*. London: Department of Health.

Department of Health (2000a) *A National Service Framework for Coronary Heart Disease*. London: Department of Health (http://www.doh.gov.uk/nsf).

Department of Health (2000b) *An Organisation with a Memory*. London: Department of Health.

Department of Health (2002a) *National Service Framework for Diabetes*. London: Department of Health (http://www.doh.gov.uk/nsf).

Department of Health (2002b). *NHS Performance Ratings and Indicators: July 2002* (http://www.doh.gov.uk/performanceratings/2002/index.html)

Ferlie, E.B. and Shortell, S.M. (2001) Improving the quality of health care in the United Kingdom and the United States: a framework for change, *The Milbank Quarterly*, 79(2): 281–315.

Freeman, T. (2002) Using performance indicators to improve health care quality in the public sector: a review of the literature, *Health Services Management Research*, 15(1): 126–37.

Gosden, T., Forland, F., Kristiansen, I.S. *et al.* (2001) Impact of payment method on behaviour of primary care physicians: a systematic review, *Journal of Health Services and Research Policy*, 6(1): 44–55.

Harrison, S. (2002) New Labour, modernisation and the Labour process, *Journal of Social Policy*, 31(3): 465–85.

Hood, C. (1995) The 'New Public Management' in the 1980s: variations on a theme, *Accounting, Organisations and Society*, 20(1): 93–110.

Hutchinson, A., Anderson, J.P., McIntosh, A., Gilbert, C.L. and Field, R. (2000) *Evidence Based Review Criteria for Coronary Heart Disease*. Sheffield: Royal College of General Practitioners Effective Clinical Practice Unit, University of Sheffield.

Josebury, H., Mathers, N. and Lane, P. (2001) Supporting GPs whose performance gives cause for concern: the North Trent experience, *Family Practice*, 18(2): 123–30.

Kaboolian, L. (1998) The new public management: challenging the boundaries of the management vs. administration debate, *Public Administration Review*, 58(2): 189–93.

Le Grand, J. (2002) Further tales from the British National Health Service, *Health Affairs*, 21(3): 116–28.

Marshall, M.N. and Davies, H.T.O. (2001) Public release of information on quality of care: how are health services and the public expected to respond?, *Journal of Health Services Research and Policy*, 6(3): 158–62.

Marshall, M., Sheaf, R., Rogers, A. *et al.* (2002) A qualitative study of the cultural changes in primary care organisations needed to implement clinical governance, *British Journal of General Practice*, 52(481): 641–5.

Mechanic, D. (2002) Improving the quality of health care in the United States of America: the need for a multi-level approach, *Journal of Health Services Research and Policy*, 7(S1): 35–9.

NHS Executive (1999) *Quality and Performance in the NHS: High-level Performance Indicators*. London: Department of Health.

Rogers, A., Campbell, S.M., Gask, L. *et al.* (2002) Some national service frameworks are more equal than others: implementing clinical governance for mental health in primary care groups and trusts, *Journal of Mental Health*, 11(?): 199–212.

Royal College of General Practitioners (2000) *Good Medical Practice for General Practitioners: Final Draft*. London: RCGP.

Salter, B. (2001) Who rules? The new politics of medical regulation, *Social Science and Medicine*, 52(6): 871–83.

Scally, G. and Donaldson, L.J. (1998) Clinical governance and the drive for quality improvement in the new NHS in England, *British Medical Journal*, 317(7150): 61–5.

Secretary of State for Health (2000) *The NHS Plan: A Plan for Investment, A Plan for Reform*, Cm. 4818–1. London: The Stationery Office.

Seddon, M.E., Marshall, M.N., Campbell, S.M. and Roland, M.O. (2001) Systematic review of studies of clinical care in general practice in the United Kingdom, Australia and New Zealand, *Quality in Health Care*, 10(3): 152–8.

Sheaff, R. (2001) *Responsive Healthcare: Marketing for a Public Service*. Buckingham: Open University Press.

Shekelle, P.G. (2002) Why don't physicians enthusiastically support quality improvement programmes?, *Quality and Safety in Health Care*, 11(1): 6.

Smith, L.F.P. and Harris, D. (1999) Clinical governance: a new label for old ingredients: quality or quantity, *British Journal of General Practice*, 49(442): 339–40.

Smith, P.C. (2002) Performance management in British health care: will it deliver?, *Health Affairs*, 21(3): 103–15.

Smith, R. (1998) All changed, changed utterly, *British Medical Journal*, 316(7149): 1917–18.

Sweeney, G., Sweeney, K., Greco, M. and Stead, J. (2001) Moving clinical governance forward: capturing the experiences of primary care group leads, *Clinical Governance Bulletin*, 2(1): 6–7.

Sweeney, G.M., Sweeney, K.G., Greco, M.J. and Stead, J.W. (2002) Softly, softly, the way forward? A qualitative study of the first year of implementing clinical governance in primary care, *Primary Health Research and Development*, 3(1): 53–64.

Wilson, T. and Neary, J. (2002) Clinical governance leads in primary care: keeping afloat, but only just, *Journal of Clinical Governance*, 10(1): 21–4.

8 Information for health

Diane Jones and David Wilkin

Introduction

> Information is the key to the modern age. The new age of information
> offers possibilities for the future limited only by the boundaries of our
> imaginations. The potential of the new electronic networks is breath-
> taking – the prospect of change as widespread and fundamental as the
> agricultural revolutions of earlier eras.
>
> (Department of Trade and Industry 1998: Foreword)

Information and information technology (IT) have occupied a key role in the
healthcare system for over 30 years and within health service policy for over a
decade. Originally, healthcare professionals collected information about
patients in an unstructured way, simply to act as an *aide-mémoire* for future
consultations. However, there have been rapid advances in technology,
including the overwhelming use of the worldwide web, which was estimated
to reach 175 million people by the end of 2001 (Department of Trade and
Industry 1998). These changes have altered the way people handle information and have had major implications for the development of information and
IT systems within the National Health Service (NHS).

Information and IT are critical to the provision of effective and efficient
health care at the level of the individual patient, the population and the health
care system. For the individual patient, the availability of information about
their history, circumstances, diagnosis, tests and previous treatments is essential to the delivery of appropriate and timely treatment. Failure to record and
communicate essential information can result in inappropriate treatment and
even death. At the population level, information on health needs, disease
patterns and health outcomes is fundamental to effective public health interventions. Effective and efficient management of the health care system as a
whole requires reliable and timely information on costs, inputs, activity and
outcomes. As the prime minister has stated, 'the challenge for the NHS is to

harness the information revolution and use it to benefit patients' (NHS Executive 1998: 5).

Within the NHS, primary care services are the usual point of first contact with patients, the point of departure for a wide range of episodic specialist services, and the providers of continuing care for most chronic illnesses. Three-quarters of the population consult a general practitioner (GP) in any one year, and most contacts between patients and the NHS are with primary and community health services. Primary care, therefore, has a key role in both the initial collection of information and the resulting flows of information within the wider health care system. General practice information systems hold the most comprehensive information about individual patients, their health and their health care. Indeed, the health record held by GPs is the only universal health record in England, which covers virtually the whole population. For these reasons alone, primary care information systems provide the foundations for a comprehensive information system for the NHS. Without sound foundations in primary care, the rest of the health information system is vulnerable to failure.

In this chapter, we first provide a brief history of the development of information systems and technology in primary care over the past two decades, review the current NHS information strategy and its implications for primary care, and highlight the role of primary care groups and trusts (PCG/Ts) in delivering information systems and technology for primary care. The second part of the chapter draws on evidence from our own research to illustrate the problems faced by PCG/Ts in information and communication, the current state of development of their information systems and technology, and the challenges facing them in meeting national targets.

The development of information systems in primary care

The development of information systems in the NHS has generally followed the organizational boundaries of the service. As the NHS has been repeatedly reorganized over the past three decades, information systems have been required to adapt to each reconfiguration, at the same time as responding to the rapid developments in IT. The NHS has developed separate information systems for hospitals, community health services, mental health services and general practice. Compared with hospital systems, primary care systems (community, mental health and general practice) have always fared less well in terms of funding. Within general practice, IT has developed more rapidly and has been better funded than other areas, such as dental, ophthalmic and pharmaceutical services.

In England, general practice computing developed rapidly during the 1980s, when funding for practice systems first became available. Many practices received free computer systems from suppliers, backed by large pharmaceutical companies, in return for data extracted from the system (Devlin 1998). Many home-grown systems also emerged, often developed by individual GPs themselves who felt that, as they understood their own needs more clearly, they would be better able to develop appropriate systems. By the late 1980s, there were literally hundreds of different systems available (Jones 1996). It was not until 1993 that standards began to be applied to general practice systems, with the introduction of the requirement for accreditation (RFA) (NHS Management Executive 1993). The introduction of standards resulted in a reduction in the number of systems available, as some suppliers dropped out of the market because of the costs of developing their systems to meet the new standards. Over the last 10 years, successive versions of the requirement for accreditation have raised the standards for general practice systems and by March 2003 there were only 17 systems accredited to RFA99, supplied by eleven companies (NHS Information Authority 2003).

Although standards for general practice clinical systems have been in place for almost 10 years, data quality and access to data have remained highly problematic. When first introduced, many systems were used primarily to handle drug prescribing and to supply data for the pharmaceutical companies. At best they were an *aide-mémoire* for GPs in their clinical work. With the rapid growth in general use of computers, the demands on general practice systems have changed enormously. Computers are no longer just tools for GPs. To deliver effective and efficient care, the whole primary healthcare team now needs to be able to access information from, and add information to, patients' clinical records. Clinicians want systems that cannot only store data and handle routine tasks, but also develop disease registers, handle electronic test results from hospital laboratories, manage appointment systems, provide access to research evidence, handle preventive recall systems and many other complex tasks. Managers need to use the data from practice-based systems to monitor quality of care, ease of access to services, expenditure and health needs. Access to the information held on practice-based systems is also increasingly necessary for the effective management of the service. However, while the data collected by these systems has expanded and changed over the past decade, the quality of data remains highly variable and problems of access to appropriate information persist.

In recent years, problems with the quality of, and access to, data within general practice have become serious obstacles to the exploitation of IT systems to improve patient care and better manage the health care system. In 1996, the Collection of Health Data in General Practice (CHDGP) project was initiated to develop and apply data standards. This project developed and promoted standards for data collection, entry and extraction to ensure more rigorous data from general practice systems (NHS Executive 1996). Building on the work of the CHDGP project, the NHS Information Authority launched the

Primary Care Information Services (PRIMIS) project in 2000. This project recognized that improving data quality was not just about setting quality standards or agreeing coding frameworks. It also involved changing the behaviour of those who use the systems. Hence the PRIMIS project provides training and support via a network of facilitators and by August 2002 there were 248 PRIMIS facilitators based in 223 primary care trusts (PCTs) (www.primis.nottingham.ac.uk).

Practice-based systems are no longer simply repositories for data; they are an essential tool for healthcare professionals. As the importance of high-quality data has become more apparent, standards have been introduced for computer systems (RFA standards) and data quality initiatives have been developed (CHDGP, PRIMIS). Furthermore, in 1996 the new NHS number, a unique identifier for all patients, was introduced and the NHS net was launched. Connection to the NHS net allows practices to access the internet, email services and the National Electronic Library for Health. Therefore, although there are still problems and issues to resolve and further developments to be made, practice-based computing has made substantial progress since the early 1990s.

In future, the new GP contract is likely to facilitate further improvements in data quality and the use of general practice systems. Proposals for the contract (NHS Confederation 2002) indicate a move towards increased use of quality indicators linked to remuneration (see Chapter 7). General practitioners will have to demonstrate that they are meeting the standards and PCTs will be responsible for monitoring standards. The key to these processes will be data generated by the computer system. Hence, GPs will need to be able to generate high-quality data to ensure they meet their contractual obligations. The new contract will thus constitute an essential driver to ensure the much-needed improvement in the quality of data entered into and retrieved from general practice systems.

Community health services data systems have evolved from the need to collect data to fulfil the Körner data requirements (Keen 1994) and, therefore, focus on collecting information about the number of contacts community-based health staff have with patients. In 1992, the NHS Information Management Group stated that most community systems were 'relatively primitive and do not support client care planning or multidisciplinary teams' (NHS Management Executive/IMG 1992: 40). Such systems were focused on performance management rather than patient care, although some have developed much further than this basic requirement.

The development of separate community health services systems means that these data are stored separately from practice-based data. This may be problematic for community health staff, who 'frequently work in isolation with their skilled efforts often fragmented and sometimes duplicated simply through poor information about what is happening to a patient' (Bellamy and

Morris 1991: 36). Mental health service systems have developed in a similar way and hospital-based data are held on yet further separate patient administration systems. Overall across the NHS, data are separated by organizational boundaries, which are often referred to as 'silos of information'. The provision of integrated patient care requires these silos to be broken down or, at the very least, systems must be designed to enable information to be exchanged effectively and efficiently between different sectors. However, breaking down established organizational boundaries and unlocking these silos is a difficult and complex task. Issues of confidentiality and security of data pose major technical challenges, but breaking down the barriers will also require changes in attitudes, behaviour and the culture of organizations.

The strategic vision for information in the NHS

The development of information systems in the NHS during the 1990s was shaped by a strategy set out in 1992 (NHS Management Executive/IMG 1992). The main aim of the strategy was to develop an infrastructure for information management and technology, including the NHS-wide network, the new NHS number and computerization of general practice. Although condemned as a failure by many commentators, the 1992 strategy nevertheless achieved at least partial success in many areas.

In 1998, the NHS set out its strategy for information management and technology in *Information for Health* (NHS Executive 1998). It described a vision for the future and a long-term strategy for achieving that vision. The centrepiece of the vision was the creation and delivery of the electronic health record, a life-long record for all patients of the NHS from cradle to grave. The electronic health record aimed to remove some of the problems associated with the separate silos of information, as it would enable healthcare professionals to access relevant patient information regardless of organizational boundaries. *Information for Health* set a host of other targets, including ensuring that all GPs were connected to NHS net and promoting the use of telemedicine and telecare. Unlike the previous 1992 strategy, it placed primary care and the general practice clinical record at the heart of its plans. However, the main problem with *Information for Health* was that it assumed a level playing field – that is, it failed to take account of the wide variations in information and IT systems across the NHS, especially in primary care. Furthermore, the strategy was written before the implementation of the latest NHS reorganization, the formation of primary care groups (PCGs) and PCTs. Table 8.1 outlines the key targets contained in *Information for Health* that relate to primary care. It also shows the deadlines for each target and the changes to these target deadlines introduced by subsequent policy guidance.

In 1999, the National Audit Office evaluated the implementation of the

Table 8.1 Key targets for primary care from *Information for Health* (IFH) (1998), *The NHS Plan* (2000), *Building the Information Core* (BIC) (2001) and *Delivering 21st Century IT Support for the NHS* (21st Century IT) (2002a)

Target (*Information for Health*)	IFH deadline	NHS Plan revised deadline	BIC revised deadline	21st Century IT revised deadline (deadlines up to 2005 'firm'; deadlines after 2005 'tentative')
Connect all computerized GP practices to NHS net	2000	2002: All GP practices connected to NHS net	31/03/01: 95% of GPs connected to NHS net 31/03/02: 100% of GPs connected	
Acute electronic patient record (EPR): 35% of all acute hospitals to have level 3 EPR All acute hospitals to have level 3 EPR	2002 2005	2004: 75% of hospitals to have EPR	Acute EPR Level 3 31/03/01: 10% 31/03/02: 35% 31/03/04: 75% 31/03/05: 100%	2005: All PCTs, NHS trusts actively implementing *elements* of EPRs 2007: EPR systems implemented in all PCTs, all hospitals
Primary and community EPR: Substantial progress in implementing integrated primary and community EPRs in 25% of health authorities	2002	2004: 50% of primary and community trusts to have EPR	Primary and community EPR 31/03/03: 25% 31/03/04: 50% 31/03/05: 100%	2010: Unified health record (with all appropriate social care information)
Full implementation at primary care level of first-generation person-based electronic health records (EHR)	2005			
Use of NHS net for appointment booking, referrals, radiology and laboratory requests/results in all parts of the country	2002	2005: Electronic booking of appointments for patient treatment	31/03/05: All bookings from GPs to outpatients or from outpatients to day case or inpatients to be made electronically 31/03/02: 60% electronic transfer of all biochemistry, haematology and microbiology test results 100% by 31/12/02 31/03/03: 100% electronic transfer of all radiology reports and discharge summaries between local hospitals and GPs	2005: National bookings service implemented 2007: National bookings service, all patient appointments, implemented
Community prescribing with electronic links to GPs and the PPA	2002	2004: Electronic prescribing of medicines		2005: National prescriptions service 50% 2007: National prescriptions service with full clinician and patient functionality 100% implemented

Telemedicine and telecare options considered routinely in all health improvement programmes	2002	2005: All health services will have facilities for telemedicine	2007: Telemedicine established in all GP surgeries 2007: Home telemonitoring (telecare) available in 20% of homes requiring it 2010: Home telemonitoring (telecare) available in 100% of homes requiring it
National Electronic Library for Health (NELH) accessible through local intranets in all NHS organizations	2002	31/03/01: 95% of all GPs using NELH	
Beacon EHR sites to have initial first-generation EHR in operation	2002		
Electronic transfer of patient records between GPs	2005		
24 hour emergency access to patient records	2005		
		March 2003: start to use SNOMED clinical terms	2007: Common clinical terms (SNOMED) implemented for all hospitals and primary care
		31/03/01: 98% of GP practices to be computerized 31/03/02: 100% of GP practices to be computerized	
		31/03/01: 90% of GP practices with LANs connected to NHS net, e.g. Desktop access 31/03/02: 100%	
			2005: Broadband access to every clinician and support staff in the NHS

earlier 1992 strategy and reviewed the plans set out in *Information for Health* (National Audit Office 1999). The National Audit Office warned of the need to learn from the failures of the 1992 strategy and emphasized the need for specific, measurable, achievable, reliable, time-related (SMART) objectives. From the outset, *Information for Health* was criticized for its vague targets and the fact that many targets were unachievable in the time-scales specified (Payne 1999; Keeley 2000; Mitchell 2000). In 2000, *The NHS Plan* (Secretary of State for Health 2000) clarified some of these targets and highlighted the poor history of investment in IT systems. *Building the Information Core* (Department of Health 2001a) further elaborated some of the targets set out in *The NHS Plan* and pushed for an increase in the pace of implementation.

In December 2001, the Information Modernization Board was established and published the *Primary Care Information Modernisation Programme* (Department of Health 2001b). This outlined some of the issues facing primary care, such as the lack of central guidance on the content of primary and community health electronic patient records. It also discussed rationalizing general practice clinical systems, which had previously been a contentious issue. The programme described the work the Board would be involved in, including the preparation of preliminary guidelines on information systems and information management for primary care organizations, and communication initiatives aimed at ensuring local activities were coordinated and good practice shared within primary care. While the publication of the *Programme* was a measure of the importance attached to developing information systems in primary care, it did not address the problem of inadequate resources, which is a real barrier to implementation. In April 2002, the Wanless Report (Wanless 2002a) highlighted the need for additional resources for information and communication technology in the NHS. In a letter to the Chancellor of the Exchequer, Wanless highlighted the importance of information and communication technology and went on to say that:

> . . . a key priority will be to invest effectively in information and communication technology. A major programme will be required to establish the infrastructure and to ensure that common standards are established. Central standards must be set and rigorously applied and the budgets agreed should be ring-fenced and achievements audited.
>
> (Wanless 2002b: 12)

To achieve real progress, Wanless (2002a) suggested that the £1.1 billion that the NHS spends each year on information and communication technology was not sufficient and should be doubled in 2003/4, eventually reaching £2.7 billion by 2007/8. However, it is unlikely that the problems of implementing integrated information systems will disappear overnight, even if this funding is made available. One of the most important resource requirements is appropriately skilled staff, a need that cannot be met instantly. Furthermore, frustration at the lack of progress on information systems and information technology targets has already seriously undermined motivation among many clinical and management staff. There is a need, therefore, to secure stakeholder support, change expectations and establish a culture of ongoing training and development for information and IT skills.

In June 2002, the NHS published yet another information strategy, *Delivering 21st Century IT Support for the NHS* (Department of Health 2002a). This national strategic programme once again reviewed, clarified and amended the deadlines contained in *Information for Health* and put it into context by relating the targets to the establishment of PCGs and their transition to PCT status. Targets were spread over a longer period, extending the implementation timetable to 2010. Furthermore, this latest strategy indicated an important shift in emphasis, from local management to 'greater central control over the specification, procurement, resource management, performance management and delivery of the information and IT agenda' (Department of Health 2002a: i). It highlighted the need to improve the leadership and direction given to IT, and combine this with national and local implementation based on ruthless standardization (Department of Health 2002a: i). Other service sectors, such as banking and retailing, apply strict standardization to ensure that all of their branches and franchises use the same systems and software. They recognize that allowing different systems would be both ineffective and inefficient. As Protti (2002) remarked recently in relation to the NIIS, 'one can have value for money or freedom of choice but not both' (p. 49). The latest strategy, therefore, represents a radical change in the development of information and IT systems in the NHS, as it emphasizes standardization rather than choice, and central rather than local decision-making.

The strategic vision for information in the NHS is one of an electronically driven service, in which information technology and information systems are core components. The centrepiece of the new national strategic programme is the development of the integrated care records service, which will incorporate the electronic health record and the electronic patient record concepts developed within *Information for Health* (Department of Health 2002b, c). The changes in the management of information and IT represent a fundamental shift, with nationally mandated systems, ruthless standardization and stronger central leadership via the Director General for IT and chief Information Officers located in each strategic health authority. However, implementation of this strategic vision presents major challenges for all NHS organizations and at all levels, from the largest hospital to the smallest, single-handed general practice. Primary care trusts will play a critical part in ensuring success as they are located at the interface between primary, community and hospital services and have a key role in the local implementation of national information and IT strategy.

The role of primary care groups and primary care trusts

The tripartite structure of the NHS (hospitals, community services, family practitioner services) and the small business culture of general practice have been major obstacles to the implementation of integrated information systems capable of meeting information needs for clinical care and supporting efficient management of the service. Until 2002, responsibility for information systems in primary care rested with health authorities, but health authorities were hampered in their attempts to develop and implement a coherent information strategy by the general practice culture of independent small businesses the many different IT systems in use, wide variations in the quality of data, restricted access to information and organizational boundaries. With the establishment of PCGs in 1999 and their subsequent development as PCTs, responsibility for information systems in primary and community care has passed to these new organizations. Although most general practices remain independent contractors, PCTs are in a stronger position than the former health authorities to develop and implement the NHS information strategy. First, they control a unified budget for three-quarters of NHS expenditure, including spending on GP infrastructure and services; this gives them the necessary leverage to set standards for information systems and data quality across all their health care providers. Secondly, although most general practices remain independent contractors, PCTs are likely to have increasing influence on practices through the allocation of funding for information and IT infrastructure and through their ability to incorporate IT quality requirements into the new GP contract. Thirdly, PCTs are responsible for quality assurance and quality improvement across primary and community services. They will therefore require access to appropriate and reliable information to discharge this responsibility. Fourthly, virtually all PCTs have taken responsibility for the provision of community nursing and other community health services, creating both the incentive and the opportunity to develop and implement an integrated information strategy for primary and community services. Lastly, the governance arrangements of PCTs mean that GPs, nurses and other health professionals are directly involved in formulating and implementing local policy. Given the responsibilities of PCTs for delivering improved primary and community services, commissioning hospital services, improving health, reducing inequalities and meeting key NHS modernization targets, information systems will be critical to their success in fulfilling these responsibilities.

The development of high-quality, integrated PCT information systems is, therefore, crucial to both the national NHS information strategy and the broader NHS modernization agenda. Primary and community health services information systems are basic building blocks in the creation of the integrated care records service. Improved access to health care, including electronic booking and telemedicine, requires information systems in primary and community services that can communicate with other parts of the NHS. Many of the standards and guidelines for improved quality of care contained in the national service frameworks require accessible and reliable information to be available in primary care.

Progress and challenges

In the remainder of this chapter, we examine how much progress PCGs, and more recently PCTs, have made in implementing the NHS IT strategy and the challenges facing them over the next few years. We draw mainly on findings from the third round of the national Tracker Survey of PCG/Ts carried out in early 2002 (Wilkin *et al.* 2002). Most of the findings we report here are derived from responses to postal questionnaires returned by the individuals in PCGs and PCTs who had lead responsibility for their organization's information management and technology (IM&T). We also include some data from interviews with PCG/T chief executives. Response rates for the third survey were 65 per cent for the IM&T questionnaire and 97 per cent for the chief executive interviews (Jones and Wilkin 2002).

Despite the current high level of computerization in general practice [98 per cent of practices were computerized by March 2001 (Department of Health 2001b)], information to support clinical care and to manage the service remains difficult to access and often of poor quality. This was reflected, in the first year that PCGs were established (1999), in the assessment by PCG chief executives of how well their information systems met their organization's information requirements (Table 8.2). Although some progress appeared to have been made by the time of the third Tracker Survey, it was evident that most chief executives were still not receiving the information they regarded as necessary to support their organization's core functions. Indeed, in two areas, information to support budget monitoring and workforce planning, fewer chief executives in 2001/2 than in 1999/2000 felt that the available information met their needs well. This may reflect the rapid increase in the responsibilities of PCG/Ts, including managing their own budgets and workforce, over the 3 years of the survey. In our view, two fundamental issues need to be addressed to correct the obvious shortcomings of current information systems. First and foremost is data quality – the accuracy, reliability, comprehensiveness and appropriateness of the information held on the various systems. The second issue is accessibility – information must be available to those who need it, when they need it and in a meaningful format.

Primary care groups and trusts are placing considerable emphasis on initiatives to improve the quality of data held in primary care. By early 2002,

Table 8.2 How well do information systems meet the PCG/Ts' needs for information to support core functions? (Chief executives)

Function	1 & 2 Poorly or not at all		3		4 & 5 Well or very well	
	1999/2000 (%)	2001/2 (%)	1999/2000 (%)	2001/2 (%)	1999/2000 (%)	2001/2 (%)
Health needs assessment	70	52	24	29	6	20
Commissioning	58	39	30	38	13	23
Monitoring service provision	63	39	23	46	14	15
Clinical governance	71	50	15	30	10	20
Budget monitoring	28	32	27	50	45	18
Workforce planning	74	75	16	19	10	6

Note: Rated on a 5-point scale from 1 'not at all' to 5 'very well'.

almost two-thirds (64 per cent) of PCG/Ts had adopted standards for data entry and extraction, compared with only 20 per cent the previous year. More than half (57 per cent) had joined the PRIMIS scheme, which supports training and development in information systems, and 41 per cent were employing PRIMIS facilitators to support practices. Increasing the use of standardized information management tools is key to the implementation of consistent quality standards for data held in general practice and improving accessibility of data. Table 8.3 shows the proportions of PCGs and PCTs where more than half of the practices were using some of the commonly available information management tools. In all cases, the use of these tools had increased between the second and third Tracker Surveys, suggesting that PCGs and PCTs recognize that investment in data quality initiatives is vital.

Making information accessible to those who need it is also partly an information technology issue. All PCG/T staff and all practices now have access to NHS net, email and the internet. This will enable staff to access the National Electronic Library for Health and allow progress to be made on achieving other targets, such as use of NHS net by GP practices for booking appointments and receiving laboratory results. However, ensuring that the information required is available and that staff are able to use it is often a much more difficult task. By 2002, all PCGs and PCTs reported that at least half of their practices were using electronic links for patient registration and 95 per

Table 8.3 Percentages of PCGs and PCTs reporting more than 50 per cent of practices using common information management tools in general practice

Information management tool	2000/1	2001/2
Read codes[a]	77	95
Data entry/extraction protocols	23	60
Disease management guidelines	14	56
Computerized prescribing protocols	29	48
MIQUEST[b]	10	44
Prodigy[c]	11	17

[a] Standard coding system for describing health problems, care and treatment.
[b] Morbidity information query export syntax.
[c] Prescribing rationally with decision support in general practice study.

cent said that at least half were using links for email. However, only 49 per cent said that half of their practices were able to receive laboratory test results electronically and none yet had telemedicine (visual electronic links between a GP practice and specialist clinic) options available for at least half of their practices. Telemedicine, albeit an important issue, is not an urgent priority compared with achieving more basic targets and developing high-quality data, which may account for the general lack of progress in this area.

Although all PCGs and PCTs now have access to NHS net and email, and half (52 per cent) have electronic links to their practices, the number that are using these to obtain information about practice activity is much smaller (Table 8.4). Such information is crucial to the achievement of targets contained in *The NHS Plan* (Secretary of State for Health 2000), such as reduced waiting times for GP appointments. Indeed, it would be almost unthinkable for any commercial organization to be unable to supply such basic information about the services it provides. By early 2002, most PCG/Ts had access to data on GP referrals and waiting times for GP appointments, but basic information about the number of GP or nurse consultations was available to only a minority of PCG/Ts. Data to support the implementation of the national service framework for coronary heart disease were being collected routinely in 82 per cent of PCG/Ts, but only 26 and 19 per cent were collecting information relating to the implementation of the national service framework for mental health and the national service framework for older people, respectively.

Moreover, despite significant progress and continuing investment in IM&T development, many PCG/T IM&T leads were not confident of their ability to meet some of the key national targets referred to above (Table 8.5). Virtually all GP practices are now connected to NHS net and the National Electronic Library for Health, but achieving these targets was largely a matter

Table 8.4 Access by PCG/Ts to information about general practice activity

	Information available by practice (%)	Aggregate information for PCG/T (%)	Information not available/don't know (%)
GP referral to specialist	73	78	23
GP use of investigations	34	34	66
GP referral to community	53	62	39
No. of GP consultations	39	39	61
No. of GP home visits	34	34	66
Practice nurse contacts	22	24	75
Waiting times for GP appointments	59	59	41
No. of out-of-hours calls	55	55	46

Table 8.5 Percentages of PCG/Ts expecting to meet the specified national targets (2001/2)

Target	Target deadline	1&2 Likely to meet target	3	4&5 Unlikely to meet target
All practices connected to NHS net	2002	89	5	7
Use NHS net for booked appointments	2002	17	38	45
Use NHS net for laboratory results	2002	54	19	28
Access to NELH	2002	82	13	5
Electronic patient record in use	2004	38	36	26
Electronic prescribing in use	2004	46	41	13
Electronic transfer of patient records	2005	33	40	28
24 hour emergency access to patient records	2005	28	44	28
Telemedicine and telecare options available	2005	23	33	45

Note: Rated on a 5-point scale from 1 'definitely will' to 5 'definitely will not'.NELH = National Electronic Library for Health.

of making the necessary connections to practice computer systems. Whether practice staff are making appropriate use of these connections is a different matter. The remainder of the targets in Table 8.5 require both progress in information technology and improvements in the quality and consistency of data. These targets are therefore more challenging. Thus, for example, the electronic transfer of patient records demands not only the installation of the necessary technology to connect sender and recipient, but also the negotiation of agreed protocols regarding who has access to confidential patient data, standards for the content of the record and standardized coding to aid retrieval. Availability and use of an electronic patient record is fundamental to achieving many of the other targets in the information strategy, but only 38 per cent of IM&T leads were confident that they would meet the deadline of having electronic patient records in use by 2004 and a quarter thought that they were unlikely to meet this target.

As described above, target dates have been subject to change since they were first published in *Information for Health*. The most recent changes were announced in June 2002 (Department of Health 2002a), after the data for the last round of the Tracker Survey had been collected. Some of these changes reflect a more realistic assessment of the capacity of primary care to achieve the targets in the time required. For example, the original deadline for achieving electronic booking of appointments, which IM&T leads were particularly pessimistic about, was first modified in July 2000 in *The NHS Plan* from 2002 to 2005 (Secretary of State for Health, 2000). In the latest guidance, this deadline is extended to 2007 for 'all patient appointments'. The target for using NHS net to access laboratory results was moved by 9 months from March 2002 to December 2002 and the target for using NHS net for radiology and discharge summaries was extended by one year to 2003. The deadlines for achieving telemedicine and telecare (home-based technology that can monitor a patient's condition and relay information back electronically to a doctor or nurse) targets have also been changed, perhaps reflecting the doubts about meeting the original target expressed by IM&T leads in our survey. Telemedicine must now be in place by 2007 (previously 2005) and telecare must be available in 20 per cent of homes needing it by 2007 and in all such homes by 2010. The target for electronic prescribing was originally 2002 but was moved to 2004 by *The NHS Plan* (Secretary of State for Health 2000); this deadline has now been extended to 2007 (Department of Health 2002a).

The most complex targets are the development of the electronic patient record and the electronic health record. The target for fully implementing the electronic health record in primary care was 2005, but this has been modified. Primary care trusts must now actively implement elements of electronic patient records by 2005, have systems fully implemented in 2007 and the unified health record, incorporating social care data, has been delayed until 2010.

At the time of the last Tracker Survey, most PCG/T IM&T leads felt that the main obstacles to progress were lack of staff and inadequate funding. Seventy-one per cent rated current staffing levels as inadequate. The recent injection of funding to support the rapid development of the NHS, including IM&T projects, contained in the Chancellor's 2002 spending review (Chancellor of the Exchequer 2002), will no doubt ease the funding problems. However, extra funding will not necessarily overcome the shortage of suitably trained staff and the need to train primary care professionals to make the best use of the information systems.

Conclusions

The creation of PCG/Ts represents a unique opportunity to develop integrated information systems for primary and community services and achieve goals set out in the national strategy. When PCGs were first established, they had few IM&T staff and were not fully engaged with the IM&T agenda. Some functions were still undertaken by health authorities, so PCGs lacked the staff, skills, funding and power to effect change. However, the abolition of health authorities as proposed in *Shifting the Balance of Power* (Department of Health 2001c) and the consequent rapid move from PCG to PCT status has had a major impact. Many IM&T staff have moved from defunct health authorities to PCTs, so PCTs now either employ more of their own IM&T staff or have contracts with IM&T staff based at other PCTs. Primary care trusts now have control over budgets previously held by health authorities and access to substantially increased resources. The Tracker Survey shows that PCG/Ts are making significant progress towards implementing the necessary electronic links, as well as making some progress towards improving data quality and accessibility. However, a gap remains between actual capacity and the expectations created by the desire to develop a world-class NHS information infrastructure. This gap is apparent in the setting of multiple targets that are not achievable within the given time-scales. It is therefore not surprising that PCG/T IM&T leads are sceptical about meeting national targets. However, it is encouraging that the latest strategy acknowledges some of these issues and may offer a more realistic way forward.

In this chapter, we have focused on IM&T in general practice because the data held in general practice systems are a fundamental building block for NHS-wide information systems. Other elements of primary care such as dentistry and pharmacy are also important, as are community health and mental health service information systems. Within the NHS it is important to break down the barriers between the silos of information that have been created by organizational barriers. However, it is also important to work closely with other agencies to access appropriate data to support patients more fully. Primary care trusts have a key role to play in ensuring that change occurs, both within NHS organizations and between the NHS and other sectors. Primary care trusts will play a central role in facilitating the implementation of the national information strategy, which should in turn support the delivery of improved healthcare for patients.

Information and information technology are critical to the provision of health care. The development of a modern infrastructure of information systems and information technology is essential to the achievement of the aspirations set out in *The NHS Plan* (Secretary of State for Health 2000). General practice systems have a particular significance, as the data collected within general practice constitute a core element of the integrated care records service. Over the past decade, there has been no shortage of strategies and implementation plans intended to deliver modern information systems across the NHS. Unfortunately, there is also no shortage of failures to meet targets and implement strategies. There have been many reasons for past failures, including a lack of clarity, unrealistic expectations, a lack of funding and repeated reorganization of the NHS (Jones and Wilkin 2003). The latest strategy set out in *Delivering 21st Century IT Support for the NHS* (Department of Health 2002a) takes account of these problems and goes some way to clarifying immediate objectives. Although it reduces the breadth of targets, it also introduces some new ones, such as delivering broadband access to all clinical and support staff by 2005. Furthermore, the development of the integrated care records service presents a highly challenging agenda. Importantly, however, the latest strategy and targets for NHS information systems are backed by a commitment to substantial new funding and radical changes in the way information and IT resources are managed within the NHS. Whether the NHS succeeds in implementing an information system fit for the twenty-first century will depend to a large extent on the organizations and individual health care professionals working in primary care and their ability to work across current organizational barriers. In September 2002, the NHS appointed a Director General for IT to ensure the implementation of the IT strategy, indicating the renewed importance of information and IT within the NHS. Within the NHS, there has been a tradition of national policy-making followed by local implementation. Local innovation has been encouraged, resulting in large differences between localities. The NHS has now recognized that it is time to move away from choice and local decision-making to a more centralized model that promises to be more effective (Department of Health 2002a).

References

Bellamy, K. and Morris, J. (1991) An IT community toolkit, *Health Service Journal*, 101: 36–7.

Chancellor of the Exchequer (2002) *Opportunity and Security for All: Investing in an Enterprising, Fairer Britain. New Public Spending Plans 2003–2006*. London: The Stationery Office.

Department of Health (2001a) *Building the Information Core – Implementing the NHS Plan*, p. 45. London: Department of Health.

Department of Health (2001b) *Information and Information Systems for Primary Care*

Organisations: Primary Care Information Modernisation Programme London: Department of Health (www.pcimb.nhs.uk).

Department of Health (2002a) *Delivering 21st Century IT Support for the NHS: National Strategic Programme*. London: Department of Health.

Department of Health (2002b) *Delivering 21st Century IT Support for the NHS: National Specification for Integrated Care Records Service – Consultation Draft*. London: Department of Health.

Department of Health (2002c) *Delivering 21st Century IT Support for the NHS: National Specification for Integrated Care Records Service – Consultation Draft Executive Summary*. London: Department of Health.

Department of Trade and Industry (1998) *Our Information Age: The Government's Vision*. London: Department of Trade and Industry.

Devlin, M. (1998) *Primary Health Care and the Private Sector*. Abingdon: Radcliffe Medical Press.

Jones, D. (1996) The national information management and technology (IM&T) strategy and its impact upon primary care, in M. Lloyd-Williams (ed.) *Proceedings of the Second International Symposium on Health Information Management Research (SHIMR)*. Sheffield: Centre for Health Information Management Research.

Jones, D. and Wilkin, D. (2002) Information management and technology, in D. Wilkin, A. Coleman, B. Dowling and K. Smith (eds) *The National Tracker Survey of Primary Care Groups and Trusts 2000/2001: Taking Responsibility*. Manchester: The University of Manchester.

Jones, D. and Wilkin, D. (2003) Information management and technology (IM&T) in primary care groups and trusts: the gap between national strategy and local implementation, *Primary Health Care Research and Development*, 4(2): 163–8.

Keeley, D. (2000) Information for health – hurry slowly, *British Journal of General Practice*, 50: 267–8.

Keen, J. (1994) Information policy in the National Health Service, in J. Keen (ed.) *Information Management in Health Services*. Buckingham: Open University Press.

Mitchell, P. (2000) IT is good at the simple things but grand strategies fail, *Health Service Journal*, 110(5696): supplement.

National Audit Office (1999) *The 1992 and 1998 Information Management and Technology Strategies of the NHS Executive*. London: National Audit Office.

NHS Confederation (2002) *The New GMS Contract – Delivering the Benefits for GPs and their Patients*. London: NHS Confederation.

NHS Executive (1996) *Collection of Health Data from General Practice: Overview*. Leeds: NHS Executive/Information Management Group.

NHS Executive (1998) *Information for Health: An Information Strategy for the Modern NHS 1998–2005*. Leeds: NHS Executive.

NHS Information Authority (2003) *National Accreditation and Procurement Process Service – Accreditation Testing: RFA 99 Current Status* (www.nhsia.nhs.uk/rfa/pages/temp.asp).

NHS Management Executive/IMG (1992) *An Information Management and Technology Strategy for the NHS in England: Handbook for IM&T Specialists*. London: HMSO.

NHS Management Executive (1993) *General Practice Computer Systems: Requirements for Accreditation*. Leeds: Information Management Group.

Payne, W. (1999) Too little, too late, *The Health Summary*, XV(10): 15–17.

Protti, D. (2002) *Implementing Information for Health: Even More Challenging than Expected?* London: Department of Health.

Secretary of State for Health (2000) *The NHS Plan: A Plan for Investment, A Plan for Reform*, Cm. 4818-I. London: The Stationery Office.

Wanless, D. (2002a) *Securing our Future Health: Taking a Long-term View*. London: HM Treasury.

Wanless, D. (2002b) *Securing our Future Health: Taking a Long-term View*, Letter to the Chancellor of the Exchequer. London: HM Treasury.

Wilkin, D., Coleman, A., Dowling, B. and Smith, K. (eds) (2002) *The National Tracker Survey of Primary Care Groups and Trusts 2001/2002: Taking responsibility?* Manchester: The University of Manchester.

9 Shifting the balance between secondary and primary care

Bernard Dowling and David Wilkin

Introduction

Since the early 1990s, there has been an attempt to raise the profile of primary care, relative to secondary care, within the overall structure of the National Health Service (NHS). This aim became manifest during the internal market under the Conservative administration before 1997, initially through the general practitioner (GP) fundholding scheme and later through the promotion of a primary care-led NHS (NHS Executive 1995a, b), and has continued under successive Labour governments since 1997. The purpose of this chapter is to examine the shifting balance of power between primary and secondary care through the mechanism of commissioning. We evaluate the evidence to date on whether primary care trusts (PCTs), and primary care groups (PCGs) before them, have had any success in expanding the influence of primary care in the planning and provision of secondary care services. The evidence covers how primary care groups and trusts (PCG/Ts) have taken responsibility for, and the influences on, their commissioning roles; the nature and extent of their commissioning activities; and the factors that appear to be associated with performance in commissioning.

Background

The NHS is characterized by a long-standing separation between GPs and hospital doctors (Honigsbaum 1979) that parallels the traditional division between primary and secondary care (Roland 1992; Boaden 1997). Before the foundation of the NHS, doctors working in fee-paying hospitals were dependent for their livelihood on receiving patients who had been referred to them by GPs. This determined the relative influence of consultants (and secondary care) and GPs (and primary care) in favour of the latter (Glennerster *et al.* 1994). The establishment of the NHS in 1948 created a system in which hospital doctors were paid salaries that were no longer directly linked to the number of patients referred to them by GPs and therefore their influence relative to GPs increased (Glennerster *et al*. 1994). Furthermore, the target NHS remuneration of GPs has customarily been lower than the salary range for consultants. Thus, despite Aneurin Bevan's original intention that the NHS should have at its foundation a powerful and high-status primary care sector, the creation of the publicly funded NHS actually shifted the balance of power within the medical profession away from GPs towards consultants (Glennerster *et al*. 1994), correspondingly raising the status of secondary care at the expense of primary care.

If one sector of a health service predominates over others, there is a danger that it will also exercise disproportionate command over resources and patient care may be influenced more by particular professional interests than considerations of maximum efficiency and effectiveness. The introduction of an internal market into the NHS in 1991 can be seen as a radical attempt to redress the balance of power. A basic principle behind the change was for secondary care to be purchased predominantly by the health authorities that had previously directly managed hospital services in the hope that, in accordance with 'textbook' economic theory, competition between providers would be generated that would motivate them to become more efficient in order to attract referrals (Secretary of State for Health 1989).

However, health authorities were not the only purchasing agency within the internal market. The GP fundholding scheme gave individual general practices the opportunity to purchase secondary care, albeit for a limited range of services. Because it was intended to provide a means by which general practice could shape and influence hospital services, the Conservative governments of the time saw this as an important mechanism for shifting the balance of power from secondary to primary care (NHS Executive 1995a, b). One rationale underlying this change was the continuing desire to reduce the overall control of hospital consultants over resources, an objective that arguably had begun with the introduction of general management in hospitals following the Griffiths report of the early 1980s (Griffiths 1983). Linked to this was a desire to relocate services from hospitals into primary care settings, for example outpatient clinics and diagnostic testing (Bailey *et al*. 1994).

As well as fundholding, other models of primary care-led purchasing also developed within the internal market. Multi-funds were groups of fundholding general practices that pooled their budgets to purchase the range of services included within the standard fundholding scheme in order to achieve economies of scale in management resources. Eighty total purchasing pilot projects were established in the mid-1990s, in which groups of general practices extended their purchasing role to a wider range of hospital and community services than those included in the standard fundholding scheme (Mays *et al*. 2001). Lastly, a range of locality commissioning groups developed collective alternatives to the fundholding model, usually working with health authorities to commission services on behalf of a specific area or population (Black *et al.* 1994).

Despite their political prominence, fundholders were marginal players in the internal market. Four-fifths of the budget for hospital and community services remained with health authorities. However, this did mean that fund-holders were able to secure changes in service provision through their con-tracts without destabilizing the local health economy. The available evidence suggests that providers were more responsive to fundholders' demands than to health authorities (Dowling 2000; Mays *et al.* 2000), and that fundholders sometimes managed to secure lower prices (Propper *et al.* 1998; Mays *et al.* 2000). However, these gains had the effect of creating a two-tier service (Dowling 1997, 1998; Mays *et al.* 2000) and may have been at the expense of health authority purchasers and, consequently, the patients of non-fundholding practices.

Evidence on the effectiveness of the various collective models of primary care-led purchasing is thinner than for fundholding. Many of the total pur-chasing pilots tended to be more effective in developing primary and com-munity services than in bringing about changes to hospital care (Mays and Mulligan 1998). Willis (1996) alleged that the gains claimed for fundholding could be achieved at lower cost through commissioning groups, but the only study that compared fundholding and commissioning groups suggested the most successful commissioning groups were those that most closely resembled fundholders (Glennerster *et al.* 1998; Mays *et al.* 2000).

From purchasing to commissioning

By the mid-1990s, the emphasis in government policy had already shifted from purchasing and contracting to the more collaborative relationship con-veyed by the term 'commissioning' (Secretary of State for Health 1996). In the early years of the internal market, it was expected that relationships between purchasers and providers would be secured by contracts rather than hierarchical, managerial commands and accountabilities (Robinson and Le Grand 1995). Contracts normally specified the activity levels, service stand-ards, collection and provision of relevant data and payment arrangements. However, in reality, such contracts were not legally binding commitments and the monitoring of whether their terms and conditions were being met was sometimes less rigorous than might be the case in a classic, private sector market.

The newly elected Labour government laid out its plans for modernizing the NHS in its 1997 White Paper, *The New NHS: Modern, Dependable* (Secretary of State for Health 1997). As explained in Chapter 1, at the heart of these plans were some important continuities with the previous government's policies, the clearest being the persisting separation between the procurement and supply of hospital services. The proposed commissioning role for PCGs and PCTs represented a strengthening of primary care-led commissioning, building on some of the advantages of the GP fundholding scheme and the various other models of collective GP commissioning (Wilkin 2002).

The shift from purchasing to commissioning is more than simply a change in language. In contrast to purchasing, commissioning places greater emphasis on cooperation between the budget holder and provider and on longer-term planning. The 1997 White Paper sought to end the lingering elements of competition and conflict in the internal market, replacing these with a culture of collaboration and partnership. Commissioning has been defined as the processes of specifying, securing and monitoring services to meet identified needs; these processes have strategic, long-term dimensions, in contrast to the short-term, operational activities associated with purchasing (Department of Health 2001a).

Commissioning is also seen as a softer and more collaborative activity than purchasing through contracts, with negotiation, trust and partnership being assigned far greater importance than the exercise of purchasing power (Ovretveit 1995). These contrasts are reflected in the less competitive language of official documentation. Documents specifying service delivery arrangements and payment terms are no longer called contracts, but service level agreements. It is expected that PCG/Ts will move towards long-term service agreements with providers, lasting at least 3 years so as to enable longer-term planning and greater stability. Commissioning can thus be characterized as the processes of planning, procuring and paying for high-quality services through partnerships between the commissioners and providers. These processes might also include negotiation, persuasion, target-setting, contractual demands, creating incentives and the monitoring of service delivery standards and patient outcomes. Commissioning should be a continuous process, whereby the agreements (or contracts) PCTs hold are compared with actual performance in delivering services on an ongoing basis to ensure the terms of those agreements are being met (Dowling *et al.* 2002). As such, while commissioning is a more collaborative process than purchasing, it does not preclude PCTs from using more aggressive market behaviour.

The continuing separation between the commissioners and the providers of hospital and other specialist services suggests that the 'new' NHS still operates as a quasi-market, albeit modified in several important respects. A quasi-market differs from a classic or conventional market in one or more of three ways. First, the agents in the exchange relationship may not necessarily seek to maximize their profits. Secondly, agencies may purchase services on behalf of the end consumers of services (patients in the case of the NHS). Thirdly, payments for services may be centralized away from the immediate purchaser or end consumer and perhaps made in the form of vouchers or other substitutes for cash (Le Grand 1991). Only the last element of this definition of a quasi-market does not feature in the exchange relationship between PCTs as commissioners and the providers of services. Hence, despite government claims that it has replaced the NHS internal market with a 'Third Way' based on longer-term partnerships and collaboration, the relationships between PCTs and other providers of services do nevertheless retain distinctive 'quasi-market' features. The partnership model of commissioning advocated by government is similar in many respects to patterns of relational contracting operated between large companies and their suppliers (such as supermarkets and food producers).

It is important to remember that commissioning is but one of the core functions of PCTs (Department of Health 1998). They are also charged with improving the health of their registered populations and reducing inequalities. Their provision of primary and community services and their commissioning of hospital services should also contribute to these wider goals through the provision of integrated, high-quality health care. Unlike the GP fundholding scheme and its variants, the commissioning of specialist services by PCTs is required to be consistent with a broader strategy for improving services, reducing inequalities and improving health. *The NHS Plan* (Secretary of State for Health 2000) and *Shifting the Balance of Power in the NHS* (Department of Health 2001b) have further strengthened the central role that PCTs are expected to play in NHS modernization. With the abolition of the health authorities in April 2002 and their replacement by 28 strategic health authorities, PCTs have taken on many of the responsibilities of the old health authorities, including full responsibility for commissioning specialist services.

How well PCTs perform in their commissioning role will be a critical factor in determining their success in improving health and health care. An important element in this will be the extent to which they are able to shift the balance of power between primary and secondary care. In the remainder of this chapter, we examine the progress made by PCGs and PCTs in taking responsibility for commissioning since the establishment of PCGs in 1999, drawing on 3 years of data from the National Tracker Survey of Primary Care Groups and Trusts (Wilkin *et al.* 2002). We examine the extent to which PCG/Ts had taken full responsibility for commissioning before the abolition of the health authorities; the influences on their commissioning priorities; commissioning activity by PCG/Ts; and possible factors that might explain differences in commissioning activity.

Taking responsibility for commissioning

With the abolition of the old health authorities in April 2002, all responsibility for commissioning hospital and specialist health services was finally devolved to PCTs. Yet the process of transferring the commissioning role from health authorities to PCG/Ts had been underway since April 1999. During the first 2 years after their establishment, PCG/Ts had limited management and administrative budgets and thus limited capacity to take on the complex process of commissioning. However, it was anticipated that they would draw on the experience and expertise of GPs and other primary care staff who had been involved in the fundholding scheme and in other models of primary care-led commissioning.

Not surprisingly, in their first year (1999/2000) commissioning was not a high priority for PCGs. Most had inherited contractual agreements with providers that had previously been negotiated by their health authorities (Malbon and Smith 1999). By the second year (2000/1), PCGs and the first PCTs were beginning to take responsibility for commissioning, with 71 per cent having taken over the commissioning of general and acute hospital services (Shipman and Banks-Smith 2001). However, only 55 per cent had taken responsibility for commissioning accident and emergency services and only 2 per cent for mental health services.

In their third year (2001/2), responsibility for commissioning most specialist services had passed from the health authorities to PCG/Ts in advance of the abolition of the health authorities in April 2002 (Figure 9.1). Apart from mental health, oncology and accident and emergency services, by early 2002 only about one-third of PCG/Ts relied on contributions from their health authorities in the commissioning of hospital and specialist services. However, only about a quarter of PCG/Ts were commissioning services independently. The majority were involved in collaborative arrangements with other PCG/Ts and with their health authorities. Some of these collaborations anticipated mergers due to take place in April 2002 as PCGs moved to trust status (see Chapter 6). It is likely that the widespread use of collaborative commissioning reflects a combination of shortages of managers with the necessary experience and expertise as well as a belief that larger commissioning units can be more effective and efficient.

Influences on commissioning priorities

The commissioning process is shaped by the priorities of the agents within the quasi-market. In principle, the priorities of commissioners should take precedence over the interests of providers. However, both commissioners and providers are subject to constraints and pressures emanating directly and indirectly from government. Although ministers and senior managers have declared their intention of shifting the balance of power closer to frontline staff and devolving decision-making to local levels, they have also put in place a host of national targets, standards and inspection processes.

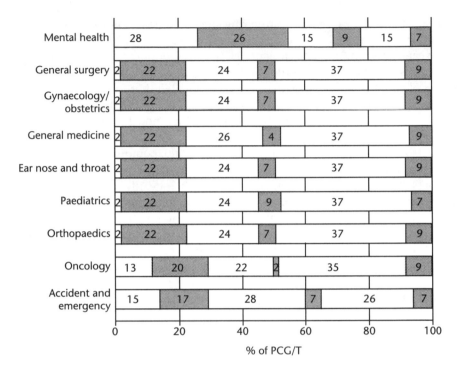

Figure 9.1 Commissioning responsibilities of PCG/Ts (2001/2). From left to right: ❏, health authority; ❏ , shared by PCG/T and health authority; ❏, this PCG/T; ❏ , another PCG/T; ❏, shared by this and another PCG/T; ❏ , this PCG/T, another PCG/T and the health authority.

Figure 9.2 shows how respondents to the national Tracker Survey in 2001/ 2 with lead responsibility for commissioning activities within their PCG/T rated the importance of a range of possible influences on the commissioning priorities of their organization. Maintaining financial balance (balancing income and expenditure), improving access to services, achieving national policy targets and implementing national service frameworks (see Chapter 7) were the key factors shaping PCG/Ts' commissioning priorities (Dowling *et al.* 2002). In other words, commissioning was predominantly influenced by national priorities and financial constraints, rather than local needs, circumstances and priorities. This perception was confirmed by the opinions of PCG/ T chief officers, many of whom perceived national targets to outweigh the importance of local priorities (Smith *et al.* 2002).

Apart from the impact of central policies on the commissioning priorities of PCTs, their ability to shape the behaviour of providers through commissioning may be further constrained by the fact that providers are performance managed by strategic health authorities, which are, in turn, predominantly concerned with national targets, policies and objectives. These performance

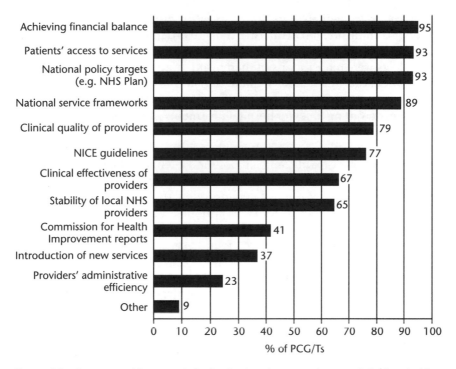

Figure 9.2   Factors rated by commissioning leads as important in commissioning decisions (2001/2). Rated 4 or 5 on a 5-point scale from 1 'very unimportant' to 5 'very important'.

management and accountability arrangements are therefore likely to give precedence to national policy priorities and objectives, at the expense of local issues. Although PCTs also appear to have prioritized national targets over local issues (see above), the direct, hierarchical managerial relationship between strategic health authorities and hospitals does potentially undermine the influence of PCTs through the commissioning process. For PCTs to succeed in shifting the balance of power towards primary care, as commissioners they are likely to need some leverage over providers.

The performance of primary case groups/trusts in service commissioning

As argued above, commissioning is the main mechanism by which PCTs can influence, shape and even determine the range and quality of hospital and specialist health services. A basic principle of quasi-market theory is that providers will be motivated to be more efficient and supply better quality services if they consider themselves to be in danger of losing business from the purchaser or commissioner (Glennerster *et al.* 1994). In theory, this renders providers more susceptible to the influences of commissioners. The fact that fundholders were more successful than health authorities in influencing hospital providers during the 1990s, through their threatened and actual capacity to move contracts to alternative, 'better' providers, led to the creation of a two-tier system of waiting times for hospital treatments (Dowling 2000). This could be interpreted as a partial shift in the balance of power to primary care. However, the contracts placed with hospitals by fundholders were small, relative to the providers' total capacity, and did not fundamentally threaten the stability of providers.

Moving contracts to a better performing (however defined) provider remains, in theory, an option for PCTs, although it is not actively encouraged because of the potential impact on the stability of providers (Secretary of State for Health 1997). The Tracker Survey found very little evidence that PCG/Ts had moved work from one provider to another. Even by their third year, only 10 per cent of PCG/Ts had changed providers for community health services. Even fewer (7 per cent) had changed their providers of mental health services; and out of the entire sample of around 70 organizations, just one PCG/T had changed its provider of hospital-based care and this only for one specialty, orthopaedics. Similarly, the value of the services that PCG/Ts have commissioned from non-NHS providers remains very small. The overwhelming bulk of their expenditure on hospital and community health services goes to existing NHS organizations (Dowling *et al.* 2002). On the basis of the evidence from the first 3 years, it is likely that the commissioning behaviour of PCTs, in terms of their willingness to change providers, will be closer to that of the old health authorities than to that of more aggressive fundholding practices.

Although the language of commissioning now uses the term 'agreement', rather than contract, agreements nevertheless still have an important role in formally defining the content and standards of services as well as the payments to be made to providers. Replacing contracts with service level agreements was intended to give a longer time scale to the agreements reached through commissioning. Initially, service level agreements would cover the same 12-month periods as the previous contracts, but it was expected that commissioners and providers would work towards long-term service agreements, usually for 3 years. This longer time scale was intended to reduce the high transaction costs associated with the former quasi-market (Secretary of State for Health 1997). However, in 2001/2 most PCG/Ts were still using one-year service level agreements. Only 17 per cent had negotiated any long-term service agreements with providers. Around half the respondents to the 2001/2 Tracker Survey thought that longer-term agreements could compromise their ability to make changes and create inflexibility, while others thought they could make relationships go stale (Dowling *et al.* 2002).

Reaching agreements with providers can also offer opportunities to set targets, create incentives and develop care pathways. In 2001/2, the Tracker Survey found that 89 per cent of PCG/Ts were setting providers targets to reduce waiting times for outpatient appointments; 26 per cent of these targets had been fully achieved and 68 per cent partially achieved. Four-fifths (79 per cent) of PCG/Ts reported setting targets to reduce waiting times for elective surgery; 29 per cent reported the targets had been fully achieved and 61 per cent partially achieved. Less success was reported by the 65 per cent of PCG/Ts that had set targets to improve hospital discharge arrangements; only 5 per cent stated that their targets had been fully achieved (although 81 per cent were partially achieved). It appears, therefore, that targets have begun to be used as a mechanism for influencing providers, an indication of the potential for PCTs to exercise leverage over secondary health care providers through the commissioning process.

Another instrument that can be used in the commissioning process to bring about improvements or changes in services is the inclusion of financial incentives within service level agreements and long-term service agreements. However, in 2001/2 only 12 per cent of PCG/Ts had done this, fewer even than the previous year when 17 per cent had done so. The majority of the incentives identified by respondents to the Tracker Survey were non-recurring bonuses to reward adherence to waiting time targets (Dowling *et al.* 2002).

A third mechanism that PCTs can use to influence and shape secondary care through the commissioning process is to incorporate quality standards into their agreements with providers. Almost a third (32 per cent) of PCG/Ts had set quality standards for acute medical care for older people, according to the 2001/2 Tracker Survey (Wilkin *et al.* 2002). Examples of quality standards included measures to ensure the acute sector supplied 28 days of any drugs required by discharged patients; improvements in discharge planning; shorter waiting times; and, most commonly, elements of the national service frameworks. National service frameworks were also mentioned frequently by the 24 per cent of PCG/Ts that had incorporated quality standards into agreements for the care of diabetic patients.

Fourthly, integrated care pathways can be agreed and incorporated into service agreements with providers. Care pathways stipulate agreed and explicit standards of care for different categories of patients and aim to specify the route through a range of health and social care services so as to provide an integrated and seamless service. They will usually specify the type of care and treatment to be provided, which professional(s) will be involved and their level of skills, and where treatment or care will take place (Department of Health 2001a). The 2001/2 Tracker Survey (Wilkin *et al.* 2002) found that, although only a minority of PCG/Ts had integrated care pathways in place for each medical specialty, virtually all PCG/Ts were in the process of developing them (Figure 9.3). However, there is no evidence

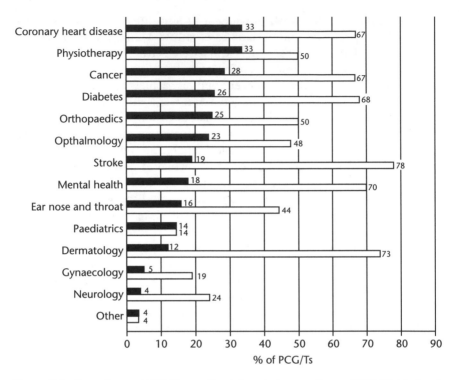

Figure 9.3 Percentages of PCG/Ts reporting integrated care pathways (2001/2). ■, already in place; ❑, planning to develop.

of the impact of these integrated care pathways on patients' experiences or outcomes.

In summary, the evidence suggests that PCG/Ts' progress in shaping hospital and specialist health services through the commissioning process has been incremental rather than radical. They have tended to concentrate their efforts on a few key areas of major concern. Moreover, although PCG/Ts see national priorities as more important influences than local concerns, even these appear to have been addressed rather unevenly and inconsistently, with some PCG/Ts being more proactive in trying to influence providers' behaviour than others.

Explaining variations

Each of the individual measures of PCG/T commissioning activity used in the Tracker Survey showed substantial variation in levels of activity between different PCG/Ts. It was clear that some PCG/Ts were much more actively engaged in using the commissioning process to improve services than others, although we have no evidence about the impact of this activity on the services received by patients. Nevertheless, it is reasonable to assume that more active PCG/Ts were more likely to generate improvements in provision than less active PCG/Ts. To explore these variations in commissioning activity, we constructed a crude indicator of commissioning activity, using answers to questions on the use of long-term service agreements, targets in commissioning, incentive schemes for providers, quality standards for specific services and integrated care pathways (Dowling *et al.* 2002).

Scores on this crude indicator of commissioning activity ranged from zero to 21 points, with higher scores representing greater activity. The highest score attained was 14 and the lowest was 1. The scores were grouped into three categories, the best performers (scores of 8 or more), average performers (scores between 3 and 7), and worst performers (scores of 1 or 2). One-fifth (20 per cent) of the sample was in the 'best performers' category, two-thirds (65 per cent) were 'average performers' and 15 per cent were 'worst performers'. Scores on this measure of activity were also reflected in commissioning leads' assessments of the leverage they had over providers. They were asked to rate their leverage over providers on a 5-point scale ranging from 'very little' (1) to 'a great deal' (5). Mean leverage scores were 3.1 for the best performing commissioners, 2.7 for average performers and 2.4 for worst performers. Perhaps not surprisingly, therefore, more active PCG/Ts felt that they exercised greater leverage over their providers (Dowling *et al.* 2002).

It might be expected that PCTs would have been more active as commissioners than PCGs. The greater autonomy of PCTs, particularly over their budgets, should in principle be associated with a more proactive approach to commissioning. Indeed, PCTs should already have shown themselves to be mature and effective organizations in order to make the transition from PCG status. The wider range of responsibilities of PCTs also means they would be likely to employ more staff that could contribute to the commissioning function and would also secure more respect from providers. However, there were no apparent differences in the commissioning performance of PCGs and PCTs (Figure 9.4). It is possible that the organizational upheaval caused by the transition to trust status, often at the same time as a merger with another PCG/T, may have diverted attention away from core functions and compromised commissioning activity, at least in the short term.

One of the arguments used to support mergers among PCG/Ts has been that their increased size should enable them to increase their capacity to engage in activities such as commissioning and increase their leverage over providers (Wilkin *et al.* 2003). Standard economic theory suggests that big purchasers or commissioners have greater market power than small

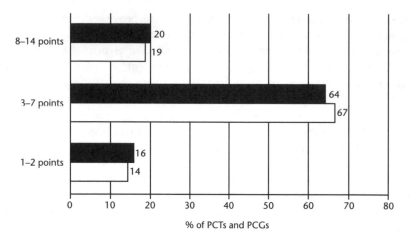

Figure 9.4 Commissioning performance of PCGs and PCTs (2001/2). ■, PCTs; ❑, PCGs.

purchasers, because providers or suppliers are more likely to be dependent on their business. On the other hand, public sector quasi-markets do not share the characteristics of many private sector markets. Consequently, large commissioners in the public sector may have a more explicit responsibility to support financially public providers, while smaller purchasers (such as fundholders) have greater freedom to pursue their own aims (Dowling 2000).

According to the Tracker Survey, larger PCG/Ts (covering populations over 200,000) did in fact perceive themselves to have more leverage over providers than the smaller PCG/Ts (Dowling *et al.* 2002). However, there is little evidence that this affected activity levels, according to the various crude indicators of performance described above. For example, nearly one-fifth (19 per cent) of the Tracker Survey's sample of PCG/Ts had populations over 200,000 in 2001/2, but that year none had introduced financial incentives into service agreements with providers, and none were using long-term service agreements. Just a single PCG/T with a population over 200,000 had introduced quality standards for acute medical care for older people, and only two had introduced quality standards for diabetic services.

Conclusions

Since early 1999, the budget and responsibility for all commissioning of hospital services has shifted from a mix of health authorities, general practice fundholders and an assortment of collective commissioning and purchasing agencies to PCTs. This alone represents a significant shift in the balance of power, as primary care no longer has the option not to 'opt in' to the commissioning process.

However, the evidence to date suggests that the change this has brought about is less than might be expected. Primary care groups and trusts have suffered from both limited capacity and experience. Many have attempted to make best use of their limited capacity by collaborating with other PCG/Ts in commissioning hospital and specialist services. One of the effects of this collaborative approach is that much commissioning has continued to be conducted at the same level, in terms of the size of population served, as the old health authorities. This brings a danger identified by Dowling (2000) as prevalent during the internal market – that the greater responsiveness and adaptability of smaller commissioners, relative to bigger ones, might be lost in the 'new' NHS.

The argument of Le Grand *et al.* (1998) that different types of services are best commissioned at different population levels is persuasive. For example, it could be argued that high-cost/low-volume services are best commissioned for large populations than low-cost/high-volume services. In short, complex tasks such as the commissioning of a wide variety of health care services may best be tackled through flexible arrangements. Primary care trusts may therefore need to be adaptable enough to commission different services for different sized populations, rather than commissioning all services for populations of around a quarter of a million people, even if this does increase transaction costs. This process should also include the devolution or centralization of budgets for commissioning to the different levels at which the commissioning takes place (Smith and Goodwin 2002).

There is little evidence that PCG/Ts have used their purchasing power to move contracts to alternative providers. This may reflect the adoption of the more collaborative model of commissioning that seems to be favoured by the Labour government, in contrast to the rather more aggressive form of purchasing often taken up by fundholders during the internal market. Definitive evidence on the impact of this new approach is not yet available. However, in 2001/2 most commissioning leads of PCG/Ts believed they had little leverage over other providers.

Commissioning secondary and specialist health services is only one function of PCTs and, indeed, may be a lower priority than developing primary and community services, a responsibility with which the professional stakeholders in PCTs are likely to be more familiar. Moreover, the high political salience of the hospital sector, including waiting lists and capital developments, has continued undiminished since the 1990s. Consequently, even if PCTs do try to exercise greater purchasing leverage, they may be constrained by the combined effect of government priorities and hospital trust accountability and performance management systems. These, in turn, threaten to undermine and marginalize PCTs' commissioning role. Nevertheless, there is

evidence that some PCG/Ts have used their new commissioning responsibilities to improve the integration of services through the development of care
pathways, provide new services and set new quality standards and targets
(Dowling *et al.* 2002).

Overall, it does not appear that the balance of power has yet shifted significantly from secondary to primary care. However, there are signs that power
may be starting to shift in line with that aim. It must also be remembered that
the growth in the power of secondary care *vis-à-vis* primary care took place,
with virtually no government intervention, over more than 40 years from the
late 1940s until the internal market began in the early 1990s. Since then, there
have been several experimental purchasing and commissioning configurations in the quest for a format most likely to redress the balance of power and
resources. If PCTs are to be successful, they are unlikely to achieve this overnight and it is perhaps unrealistic to expect radical change so soon. Hence the
key to shifting the balance of power towards primary care may lie in a period of
structural stability, so that PCTs have both the time and resources to do what is
expected of them.

References

Bailey, J., Black, M. and Wilkin, D. (1994) Specialist outreach clinics in general
practice, *British Medical Journal*, 308(6936): 1083–6.
Black, D., Birchall, A. and Trimble, I. (1994) Non-fundholding in Nottingham: a
vision of the future, *British Medical Journal*, 309(6959): 930–2.
Boaden, N. (1997) *Primary Care: Making Connections*. Buckingham: Open University
Press.
Department of Health (1998) *A First Class Service: Quality in the New NHS*. London:
Department of Health.
Department of Health (2001a) *National Service Framework for Older People: Modern
Standards and Service Models*. London: Department of Health.
Department of Health (2001b) *Shifting the Balance of Power in the NHS: Securing
Delivery*. London: Department of Health.
Dowling, B. (1997) Effect of fundholding on waiting times: database study, *British
Medical Journal*, 315(7103): 290–2.
Dowling, B. (1998) Potential biases do not affect results of waiting times study,
British Medical Journal, 317(7150): 79.
Dowling, B. (2000) *GPs and Purchasing in the NHS: The Internal Market and Beyond*.
Aldershot: Ashgate.
Dowling, B., Coleman, A., Wilkin, D. and Shipman, C. (2002) Commissioning, in
D. Wilkin, A. Coleman, B. Dowling and K. Smith (eds) *The National Tracker
Survey of Primary Care Groups and Trusts 2001/2: Taking Responsibility?* Manches-
ter: The University of Manchester.

Glennerster, H., Matsaganis, M. and Owens, P. with Hancock, S. (1994) *Implementing GP Fundholding: Wild Card or Winning Hand*. Buckingham: Open University Press.

Glennerster, H., Cohen, A. and Bovell, V. (1998) Alternatives to fundholding, *International Journal of Health Services*, 28(1): 47–66.

Griffiths, R. (1983) *NHS Management Enquiry*. London: Department of Health and Social Security.

Honigsbaum, F. (1979) *The Division in British Medicine: A History of the Separation of General Practice from Hospital Care 1911–1968*. London: Kogan Page.

Le Grand, J. (1991) Quasi-markets and social policy, *The Economic Journal*, 101(408): 1256–67.

Le Grand, J., Mays, N. and Dixon, J. (1998) The reforms: success or failure or neither?, in J. Le Grand, N. Mays and J. Mulligan (eds) *Learning from the NHS Internal Market: A Review of the Evidence*. London: King's Fund.

Malbon, G. and Smith, J. (1999) Commissioning, in D. Wilkin, S. Gillam and B. Leese (eds) *The National Tracker Survey of Primary Care Groups and Trusts: Progress and Challenges 1999/2000*. Manchester: The University of Manchester.

Mays, N. and Mulligan, J. (1998) Total purchasing, in J. Le Grand, N. Mays and J. Mulligan (eds) *Learning from the NHS Internal Market: A Review of the Evidence*. London: King's Fund.

Mays, N., Mulligan, J. and Goodwin, N. (2000) The British quasi-market in health care: a balance sheet of the evidence, *Journal of Health Services Research and Policy*, 5(1): 49–58.

Mays, N., Goodwin, N., Malbon, G. and Wyke, S. (2001) Health service development: what can be learned from the UK total purchasing experiment?, in N. Mays, S. Wyke, G. Malbon and N. Goodwin (eds) *The Purchasing of Health Care by Primary Care Organizations: An Evaluation and Guide to Future Policy*. Buckingham: Open University Press.

NHS Executive (1995a) *Developing NHS Purchasing and GP Fundholding: Towards a Primary Care-led NHS*. London: Department of Health.

NHS Executive (1995b) *General Practice Fundholding: A Primary Care Led NHS*. London: Department of Health.

Ovretveit, J. (1995) *Purchasing for Health: A Multidisciplinary Introduction to the Theory and Practice of Health Purchasing*. Buckingham: Open University Press.

Propper, C., Wison, D. and Söderlund, N. (1998) The effects of regulation and competition in the NHS internal market: the case of general practice fundholder prices, *Journal of Health Economics*, 17(6): 645–73.

Robinson, R. and Le Grand, J. (1995) Contracting and the purchaser–provider split, in R. Saltman and C. von Otter (eds) *Implementing Planned Markets in Health Care*. Buckingham: Open University Press.

Roland, M. (1992) Communication between GPs and specialists, in M. Roland and A. Coulter (eds) *Hospital Referrals*. Oxford: Oxford University Press.

Secretary of State for Health (1989) *Working for Patients*. London: HMSO.

Secretary of State for Health (1996) *The National Health Service: A Service with Ambitions*. London: The Stationery Office.

Secretary of State for Health (1997) *The New NHS: Modern, Dependable*. London: The Stationery Office.

Secretary of State for Health (2000) *The NHS Plan: A Plan for Investment, A Plan for Reform*. London: The Stationery Office.

Shipman, C. and Banks-Smith, J. (2001) Commissioning, in D. Wilkin, S. Gillam and A. Coleman (eds) *The National Tracker Survey of Primary Care Groups and Trusts 2000/2001: Modernising the NHS?* Manchester: The University of Manchester.

Smith, J. and Goodwin, N. (2002) *Developing Effective Commissioning by Primary Care Trusts: Lessons from the Research Evidence*. Birmingham: The University of Birmingham.

Smith, K., Coleman, A., Dowling, B. and Wilkin, D. (2002) Organizational development and governance, in D. Wilkin, A. Coleman, B. Dowling and K. Smith (eds) *The National Tracker Survey of Primary Care Groups and Trusts 2001/2: Taking Responsibility?* Manchester: The University of Manchester.

Wilkin, D. (2002) Primary care budget holding in the United Kingdom National Health Service: learning from a decade of health service reform, *Journal of the Australian Medical Association*, 176(9): 539–42.

Wilkin, D., Coleman, A., Dowling, B. and Smith, K. (eds) (2002) *The National Tracker Survey of Primary Care Groups and Trusts 2001/2: Taking Responsibility?* Manchester: The University of Manchester.

Wilkin, D., Bojke, C., Coleman, A. and Gravelle, H. (2003) The relationship between size and performance of primary care organizations in England, *Journal of Health Services Research and Policy*, 8(1): 11–17.

Willis, A. (1996) Commissioning – the best for all, in P. Littlejohn and C. Victor (eds) *Making Sense of a Primary Care-led NHS*. Oxford: Radcliffe Medical Press.

10 Improving local health

Stephen Peckham

Introduction

Since the election of the Labour government in 1997, there has been a greater emphasis on public health and the need to address the problems of health inequalities. The government's plans for the improvement of public health in England were set out in its 1997 White Paper *The New NHS: Modern, Dependable* (Secretary of State for Health 1997), a Green Paper on public health (Secretary of State for Health 1998) and the subsequent White Paper *Saving Lives: Our Healthier Nation* (Secretary of State for Health 1999). The government's strategy includes action at the national, local and individual levels, with targets for improving health, and establishing frameworks for activities in specific settings, such as schools, workplaces and local communities. These aims are also reflected in similar policies for Northern Ireland, Scotland and Wales.

In England, primary care groups and trusts (PCG/Ts) have been given an explicit responsibility to improve the health of, and to address health inequalities in, their communities (Secretary of State for Health 1997). With the dissolution of health authorities primary care trusts (PCTs) now have their own directors of public health and public health workforce (Secretary of State for Health 2000; Department of Health 2002a).

In this chapter, I outline current policy and organizational developments relating to primary care and public health in England. I then briefly review recent research on the development of public health in primary care groups (PCGs) and PCTs, drawing on national and local research. Finally I discuss the potential for a primary care-based approach to public health. The chapter draws on data from the Tracker Survey (Wilkin *et al.* 2002), research undertaken in conjunction with the UK Public Health Association on public health and primary care (Taylor *et al.* 1998; Peckham and Godel 2001) and other recent studies on the public health role of PCG/Ts.

Public health and health improvement

Within the National Health Service (NHS), the most common definition of public health is that set out in the Acheson Report (Department of Health and Social Security 1988), which examined the role of public health within the service. The report adopted the widely used World Health Organization definition of public health as the science and art of preventing disease, prolonging life and promoting health through organized efforts of society. The Abrams Committee also endorsed this definition 5 years later (Department of Health 1993). In practice, different people have different definitions and perspectives on what public health is and what its scope is (Taylor *et al.* 1998; Meads *et al.* 1999; Heller 2002).

Organizationally, the history of public health is also complex (Lewis 1986; Baggott 2000), with responsibilities split between the NHS and local authorities. Until 1974, public health services such as community medicine and health visiting were located within local authorities. In 1974, medical public health and nursing were transferred to NHS health authorities and community health services, while environmental health services remained in local authorities alongside housing, social services, leisure services and education. Public health is now undergoing another organizational transition, with a greater role for primary care and an emphasis on partnerships between local authorities and health care services through health action zones, local strategic partnerships, healthy living centres, urban and neighbourhood renewal and, in England, the development of a public health role for PCTs.

The government has defined several core functions for PCG/Ts; these include improving population health and reducing health inequalities. The government has given no precise definition of health improvement: it is referred to both in narrow terms as an NHS activity (although often distinguished from developing primary and community services and commissioning hospital care) and in broader terms to include non-NHS activities such as health promotion in schools and wider initiatives tackling the social, economic and environmental influences on health. Within PCG/Ts, health improvement is generally defined very broadly and may include NHS core activities such as providing primary care, commissioning, improving quality, improving access, strategy and prioritization (Abbott *et al.* 2001). Before exploring how PCG/Ts are tackling public health and local health improvement, it is useful to examine the policy context within which they operate.

Policy and guidance on public health and primary care groups/trusts

Since 1997, policy guidance in England has identified the need for PCGs and, subsequently, PCTs to work with other local partners, including local authorities and housing agencies, to adopt community development approaches to reach local people, to develop more one-to-one health promotion interventions, and to work with all local stakeholders to address local health issues. With the establishment of PCGs, the overall lead for public health remained with health authority directors of public health, but PCGs were required to assess local public health capacity and develop a public health perspective to address local health needs (Secretary of State for Health 1997). The public health responsibility of PCG/Ts was underlined in the *Saving Lives: Our Healthier Nation* White Paper that outlined the centrality of the health improvement programme and the important role to be played in the development of local health improvement programmes by PCGs; over time 'they will forge powerful local partnerships with local bodies . . . to deliver shared health goals. They will help shape the health improvement programme and draw up their own plans for implementing it and for hitting the targets in it' (Secretary of State for Health 1999: 122).

These changes placed an emphasis on the role of PCG/Ts in public health, which in turn, raises important questions about the appropriate roles and responsibilities of the public health workforce, of existing primary care staff and of other local workers. These questions were partly addressed by the report of the Chief Medical Officer (2001) on the need for a multidisciplinary public health workforce. This report recognized the public health role of primary care staff as well as other people working in local authorities and the wider community. With the transition of PCGs to PCTs, the government announced in 2001 the intention of integrating public health functions within PCTs, with the new strategic health authorities retaining a performance management and review role (Department of Health 2001a, 2002a).

This constitutes a major reorganization of public health responsibilities within the NHS. It presents challenges for PCTs in managing a more diverse workforce, in developing new relationships and partnerships with other organizations, and in testing the boundaries of professional expertise. *Shifting the Balance: Next Steps* (Department of Health 2002a) contained explicit guidance on the development of public health activities within PCTs. Each PCT was to have a strong public health team 'engaged with local communities, local authorities and non-Governmental agencies and focussed on improving health, preventing serious illness and reducing health inequalities in the populations they serve' (Department of Health 2002a: 18). Each PCT would have a director of public health. However, in an important change to the previous health authority-based arrangements, PCT directors of public health were no longer required to be medically qualified, although they must have a specialist public health qualification. This change follows wider trends towards a multidisciplinary public health workforce (Chief Medical Officer 2001). Primary care trusts were required to develop broad partnerships and promote the participation of their local communities. They need to work closely with local authorities, who now have a statutory duty to promote the health and well-being of their residents, have a new power of scrutiny over local NHS activities and organizations (see Chapter 11), and are responsible for developing local strategic partnerships (Department of Health 2001a). Primary care trusts were expected to become key members of local strategic partnerships and this embeds much of their public health role within an inter-agency framework – again a new approach for primary care.

A major theme of the government's approach to public health has been the renewed emphasis on tackling health inequalities (see Chapter 4). The government's strategy aims to improve the health of the population as a whole and to improve the health of the worst-off in society, in order to narrow the 'health gap'. In addition to the four targets relating to heart disease and stroke, accidents, cancer and mental health set out in *Saving Lives: Our Healthier Nation* (Secretary of State for Health 1999), two national health inequality targets, relating to life expectancy and infant mortality, have also been set (Department of Health 2001b). There are further inequality targets relating to reductions in smoking and teenage pregnancy. In England, the role of primary care is central to tackling such inequalities, with an emphasis on getting appropriate PCT arrangements in place, empowering communities, improving access to primary care services and promoting local strategic partnerships (Department of Health 2002a). However, concerns have been raised about the extent to which PCTs will actually give priority to tackling health inequalities, their capacity to take on public health issues and their capacity to change from service-led to needs-led agencies (Department of Health 2002a).

Public health and primary care

Despite sharing common roots in the nineteenth century (Lewis 1986; Baggott 2000; Peckham and Exworthy 2002), developing a public health role within primary care organizations today remains a key challenge. For many practitioners, the roles of patient advocate, mediator and population planner may overlap and conflict with one another (Pratt 1995). Research has also identified several problems in developing a public health role in primary care. Taylor *et al.* (1998) highlighted a number of barriers, including:

- The lack of a 'shared language' – common definitions of public health – between primary care practitioners and other stakeholders, including members of the community.
- A poor understanding and history of collaborative working, both within primary health care teams and between general practitioners (GPs) and other agencies.
- The dominance of a medical model of primary care with its emphasis on general practice, and medically dominated organization and values.
- Poor understanding of the key principles of public health among primary care professionals.

Meads *et al.* (1999) examined early PCGs and identified several organizational barriers to developing public health in primary care. These included the need for primary care organizations to:

- develop a public health perspective;
- acquire public health skills;
- develop organizational links with local authorities and local communities;
- develop organizational capacity.

Meads *et al.* (1999) also concluded that primary care organizations needed to change their outlook. 'Primary care groups are a fundamental "mindset" change for individuals as well as organizations. The biggest obstacles are attitudinal not structural' (health authority director of public health quoted in Meads *et al.* 1999: 47). Popay (2001) has argued that developing a public health function in PCTs places an expectation on them to deliver the public health agenda and to address inequalities in health, when there is little if any evidence from previous research or practice that primary care organizations or primary care medical professionals have the capacity or the inclination to do this. Moreover, many GPs have a very narrow view of health promotion, are often untrained in this particular field and have limited experience of community development activities. Many also have an animosity to social interventions such as health promotion, particularly if such activities compromise their traditional caring role (Macdonald 1992; Taylor *et al.* 1998; Fitzpatrick 2001).

Moreover, if the causes of health inequalities are related to wider socioeconomic or environmental factors such as income inequality and relative deprivation (Wilkinson 1996), clarity is needed about the role that primary care can play in achieving local and national health inequality targets. In relation to primary care, equity has traditionally been viewed in terms of access to, or provision of, services (Goddard and Smith 2001; see also Chapter 4). This emphasis on service provision is reflected in calls for better monitoring of inequalities in primary care, particularly in relation to the 'inverse care law' (Tudor-Hart 1988), the distribution of GPs and other health care professionals, or the size of GPs' patient lists (Smeeth and Heath 1999). While Starfield (1998) has argued that a robust primary care infrastructure has the potential to redress broader health inequalities, it is not clear what role PCTs should play or what strategies and activities they should develop. At a basic level, these could include health surveillance, regular check-ups and reviewing medical records, an approach that was advocated, and adopted, by Tudor-Hart (1988). Addressing health inequalities could also require key divisions in society to be addressed, such as social demography (age, area of residence, gender and ethnicity/race), social and economic status (car ownership, employment, income, occupational social class, socio-economic groupings, tenure status) and social environment (housing conditions, social networks and social support) (Braham and Janes 2002; Carr-Hill and Chalmers-Dixon 2002). This represents a complex agenda for PCTs to deal with and one that clearly cannot be tackled by them alone.

The challenges presented by this agenda have been recognized by the government in *The NHS Plan* (Secretary of State for Health 2000), which notes that the wider inability to forge effective partnerships with local government, business and community organizations has inhibited the NHS's ability to prevent ill-health and tackle health inequalities. This inability is perhaps most marked in general practice which, while having a poor record of partnership working (Taylor *et al.* 1998; Meads *et al.* 1999; see also Chapter 12), nevertheless provides the basic organizational building block of PCTs. In the remainder of this chapter, I review progress towards the development of a public health function within PCTs in England. (The focus is mainly on PCTs because of the relatively recent development and clarification of their public health responsibilities alongside their transition from PCG status.) I explore relevant aspects of PCTs' organizational development and public health capacity, the provision of public health services, and identify those factors that appear to support or inhibit PCTs' capacity as public health agents to improve health and reduce health inequalities.

Primary care trusts and the public health function

Research in London has shown that there is a problem in defining the public health function, with PCTs often wanting greater clarification of what this role involves (Petchey 2002). This lack of clarity is linked to the problems of defining public health, an issue that is far from new and is particularly complex in the context of primary care (Taylor *et al.* 1998; Levenson and Johnson 2000). This, in turn, creates problems in defining and developing the public health roles of primary care staff (Wirrmann 2002).

As yet there is little data on the structure of public health services within PCTs, but current guidance suggests that public health should be a responsibility of all PCT staff. This point is underlined by recent research on public health in London PCTs (Petchey 2002). This research concluded that PCTs need to recognize and build on the public health contributions of all primary health care team members. However, the lack of clarity about what constitutes public health activity and the public health roles of primary care practitioners remains (Wirrmann 2002). In practice, certain groups of PCT staff, such as health visitors, school nurses, health promotion specialists and qualified public health specialists, do already include elements of public health activities among their responsibilities. Yet the organization of such staff groups is not uniform. In Wiltshire, for example, health visitors and health promotion specialists are not employed by the local PCTs but work within a separate, special trust and are 'attached' to PCTs.

In a survey of key local public health stakeholders, Woodhead *et al.* (2002) found that respondents felt that devolution of public health responsibilities to PCTs would make this expertise more available to the community. However, although there was scope for a more effective utilization of public health expertise at local level, shortages of staff with appropriate expertise was currently a potential drawback. Public health professionals participating in a joint NHS Leadership Centre and Faculty of Public Health Medicine meeting to explore leadership issues echoed these points. Moving public health to PCTs was seen as beneficial, as it was felt that this would enhance local sensitivity, improve working with local government, involve frontline workers more, focus more on the wider determinants of health and bring new skills and non-medical perspectives. However, concern was also expressed about the isolation of public health staff working within PCTs, the replication of functions across many agencies, the large and varied agenda, the small size of PCTs and the loss of corporate memory through the fragmentation of public health departments that had been built up in the former health authorities (Scott 2002).

Currently, PCTs are only just developing their public health staff groups. While government policy does not require a PCT director of public health to be medically qualified, most are public health doctors who have moved from the old health authority public health departments. In March 2003, of the 313 PCTs with directors of public health, 283 had made director appointments while 30 had acting appointees. Of the 283 appointed, 234.5 (83 per cent) were medically qualified and 48.5 (17 per cent) were non-medics (M. Tagney, Department of Health, personal communication). However, the distribution of medical and non-medical appointments has not been even. For example, in the London region only four of the 32 PCTs had non-medically qualified directors of public health and in the southwest seven of 42 and in the east midlands only two of 26 directors were non-medics. This contrasts with northwest England, where 15.5 of the 42 appointed directors are non-medics (including one medic/non-medic job share), and with northeast England, where five of 14 directors are non-medics.

There are two possible reasons for this pattern. First, there was the need to place the former health authority public health specialists in new positions. Medical specialists dominated the health authority public health departments, so there was a larger pool of medical than non-medical public health specialists, especially at consultant and director of public health levels, seeking new positions. Second, despite moves towards multidisciplinary public health, it is still very much a medically dominated profession working to medical models. It therefore remains difficult for non-medical public health specialists to gain a foothold. In contrast, in northwest England, there has been a specialist public health training scheme open to all public health staff for some time, thus creating a larger non-medical pool of suitably qualified and experienced staff from which to appoint PCT directors of public health.

Each PCT is intended to be part of a network of public health skills, knowledge and experience, 'to enable the provision of public health expertise which cannot be provided in every PCT but can be made available through the network' (Department of Health 2002a: 18). However, there is little guidance on how such networks should be developed. The aim was that they should be 'bottom-up', involving a range of representatives from statutory and non-statutory agencies within the local community, but guidance from the government (Department of Health 2002a) and professional bodies (Faculty of Public Health and Health Development Agency 2001) advocates the establishment of professional-only networks. This was clearly the case in one of the UK Public Health Association (UKPHA) research case studies, where there was a complete detachment of the newly established Public Health Network from existing voluntary, local government and professional networks in the PCT area, including one network specifically responsible for addressing health inequalities. In fact, the public health consultant mandated to establish the network had no knowledge of other existing groups (unpublished field notes, UKPHA study). This lack of clarity is causing some inertia in areas without existing developed networks upon which a wider public health network can be built. It is intended that directors of public health should lead these networks, which will bring together public health specialists and practitioners across the NHS and local government (Faculty of Public Health and Health Development Agency 2001). The danger is that new professional, or expert, networks could be established that will displace, or even ignore, existing networks or partnerships that have been addressing public health issues. It is also not clear how a wider public health workforce, including workers in the voluntary and community sector and community activists, will be drawn into such networks; this is an issue I return to later in the chapter.

The Tracker Survey found that by 2001/2, 68 per cent of PCG/T boards had a subgroup responsible for health improvement and 84 per cent had a designated health improvement lead person (Gillam and Smith 2002). It is not yet known how many PCTs have established public health networks. Nor is it yet clear how many PCTs have fully established their public health teams – the minimum recommended by the Faculty of Public Health Medicine is one director, two whole time specialists (one non-medical and one medical), three health promotion specialists and a public health intelligence officer. There is a clear feeling among public health specialists and other members of PCTs that public health is still a very new function for PCTs. One PCT director of public health commented that he felt very isolated, with too many demands being placed on too few resources:

> I am constantly being asked to attend meetings with outside groups, engage with other agencies, meet community organizations and participate in the management of the PCT . . . This is too much for one person. How do I decide what is of real value?
>
> (Unpublished field notes, UKPHA study)

Although other PCT staff share these pressures, they could explain why fewer public health specialists are engaged in more central PCT issues such as quality improvement; only 35 per cent of public health professionals are reported to be involved in clinical governance (Gillam and Smith 2002). Heller (2002) found that staff in PCTs felt they had very basic requirements for developing their public health roles. These included wanting more information about preventive measures, health needs assessment and evidence-based practice to guide informed decision-making to improve health. There was also concern about the quality, quantity, accuracy and relevance of the information that was available. For example, 'one in five (20 per cent) of chief executives reported that the information they received to support needs assessment was not actually meeting these needs at all, an increase on previous years (7 per cent in both 1999/2000 and 2000/01)' (Gillam and Smith 2002: 106).

Establishing a public health function within PCTs is a recent development, with director appointments and a wide range of organizational development issues still to be addressed. Research (Heller 2002; Petchey 2002) has found that PCT representatives have clear ideas about the development of a public health role, with an emphasis on approaches that are locally based, operational (rather than strategic) and 'mainstreamed' within the organization, not simply delivered by a small group of 'public health professionals'. 'Mainstreaming' raises multiple challenges and numerous skills gaps have been identified among staff in primary care, especially among nurses, GPs and ancillary staff (Burke *et al.* 2001). However, PCG/Ts have been required to address public health issues since their creation in 1999 and it is useful to review this experience. In the next section, therefore, I examine the existing evidence on the extent to which PCG/Ts have engaged in health improvement activity.

Primary care trusts and local health improvement

Despite the complexities of developing organizational structures for public health within PCTs and across inter-agency and local community partnerships, the test of PCT public health activity is the extent to which it contributes to local health improvement. However, while PCG/Ts are discrete organizations with identifiable structures, there are also enormous variations between their constituent parts, reflecting wide differences between general practices, primary health care teams and community health services, not to mention their social care and partnership arrangements. Similarly, the public health activities that each of these constituent parts of the PCG/T might undertake will be varied and might include interventions by individual practitioners, multidisciplinary groups such as primary care teams or general practices, specialist initiatives employing project-specific staff such as community health development or smoking cessation, and multi-agency/partnership groups working with practitioners from other agencies. Additionally, PCTs can adopt structural approaches through their corporate activities and policies, including their employment and purchasing policies and healthy workplace initiatives.

Most PCTs have strengthened their strategic planning capacity in support of health improvement, a process required specifically in the transition from a PCG. They have also identified local priorities and some can point to evidence of implementation in addressing health inequalities. For example, the 2001/2 Tracker Survey (Gillam and Smith 2002) found a substantial increase in local health needs assessment activity, with 82 per cent of PCG/Ts reporting having their own health improvement programme (compared to 73 per cent the previous year). Nearly all (92 per cent) PCG/Ts had designated a board or executive committee member with specific lead responsibility for health improvement, and there was a clear trend towards appointing public health specialists to PCG/Ts (an increase from 14 per cent in 2000/1 to 43 per cent in 2001/2). Interestingly however, there was also an increase (from 9 per cent in 2000/1 to 20 per cent in 2001/2) in the proportion of PCG/Ts designating a nurse as the health improvement lead board/executive committee member, suggesting that some PCG/Ts do not automatically see medical public health doctors as the natural leads (Gillam and Smith 2002). In addition, 67 per cent of PCG/Ts had set health improvement targets; just over half had targets for reducing smoking, 43 per cent for reducing teenage conception rates and a third for reducing differences in life expectancy (Gillam and Smith 2002). The extent of these health inequality targets contrasted with the previous years, when the Tracker Survey had found that levels of activity to address health inequalities remained low and that the strategies in use needed to be expanded (Gillam and Smith 2002).

Clearly, public health activities of different kinds have always been undertaken by primary health care team members and within GP practices, and developments throughout the 1980s and 1990s aimed to extend and develop these roles. Such approaches have been reviewed elsewhere (NHS Centre for Reviews and Dissemination 1995; Ashenden *et al*. 1997; Hulscher *et al*. 2001). The remainder of this section deals predominantly with the activities of PCG/ Ts in five areas: supporting individual approaches by practitioners; as members of public health partnerships; supporting special public health projects; organizational approaches; and working with local communities.

Individual approaches to public health

Primary care groups and trusts have supported and developed health promotion activities undertaken by practitioners. Much of this is secondary and tertiary prevention (see Chapter 4) and concerns key health improvement priorities, such as reducing coronary heart disease or smoking (Butler *et al*. 1998; Lennox *et al*. 2001) and improving diabetes care. These activities reflect the priorities set by PCG/Ts in their health improvement strategies (Gillam and Smith 2002). Research has also shown that GP advice on child safety, coupled with the provision of low-cost safety equipment for families on means-tested benefits, leads to increased use of equipment and other safe practices (Clamp and Kendrick 1998).

There is also evidence that opportunistic GP advice to stop smoking is an effective way of reducing smoking rates (Butler *et al*. 1998). Approaches such as these suggest that there is much primary care can do to address inequalities in health, especially if this is linked to wider social interventions, such as increasing income for people on benefits or providing appropriate advice and support on specific health issues. The PCG/Ts have supported smoke-stop projects and are beginning to examine differences between GP practices in take-up rates for cervical screening and immunization, through their clinical governance procedures (see Chapter 7).

However, although official policy and guidance identifies the wider primary health care team as being part of the public health workforce (Burke *et al*. 2001; Chief Medical Officer 2001), practitioners themselves have different, and often contradictory, views about what constitutes public health and what their role in this is. For example, GPs have traditionally focused on individual, reactive, medical care (Pratt 1995; Taylor *et al*. 1998) and many do not see a public health role for themselves (Fitzpatrick 2001). In addition, recent research exploring the public health role of nurses suggests that practice nurses and district nurses see public health as someone else's role, with their own contributions lying mainly in patient care or individual health education (Wirrmann 2002).

Primary care groups/trusts and public health partnerships

As outlined above, central to current developments to tackle inequalities and secure health improvement is the notion of partnership with local communities, local authorities and other agencies (see also Chapter 12). The Local Government Act 2000 placed a duty on local authorities to prepare community strategies that set out their plans to promote the economic, social and environmental well-being of their areas. Each local area is required to have a local strategic partnership that brings together the public, private, voluntary and community sectors to implement the local community strategy. These developments are located within the broader framework set by the Act, which is aimed at the modernization of local government and local democratic renewal. Local strategic partnerships are intended to bring together all other local inter-sector partnerships (Department of Environment, Transport and the Regions 2000, 2001), engaging communities in partnership arrangements and rationalizing other strategic planning processes. Tackling health inequalities is a central focus for these partnerships and PCTs are seen as important partnership members bringing knowledge, expertise and resources to the partnership (Department of Health 2001b).

However, there are fears that local strategic partnerships are being dominated by local authorities with little community input (Biles *et al.* 2001); respondents in our UK Public Health Association research were also concerned that health improvement programmes currently remain separate from the community plans being developed by local authorities. There does not appear, at present, to be any significant dovetailing of NHS planning with these new local strategic partnerships. Yet public health, in its broadest terms, is clearly expected to be a prominent issue for local strategic partnerships. The building of such alliances was a key recommendation of the NHS Centre for Reviews and Dissemination (1995) report on variations in health.

By 2001/2, all PCG/Ts were involved in partnerships with local authority departments to improve health, with 100 per cent working in partnerships relating to community development and regeneration activities and 35 per cent on welfare rights programmes (Coleman and Glendinning 2002). The PCG/Ts are also increasing their involvement in wider multi-agency activities. The most common activities in 2001/2 were SureStart (85 per cent) and leisure services (73 per cent) (Gillam and Smith 2002).

For example, in one locality in southern England, the health improvement subgroup of the PCG board grew from an existing health action partnership and was chaired by the local authority health policy officer (Hudson *et al.* 1999). In other areas, new partnerships are also developing well. In Croydon, for example, there is coterminosity between all major agencies, both statutory and non-statutory. The Croydon Strategic Partnership Board oversees themed areas of work and the health improvement programme comes under the Healthy Croydon Partnership, one of these themed areas, with sections written and agreed by supporting joint planning teams (Hamer and Easton 2002).

There have also been recent trends towards the joint funding of specialist public health posts. Although many of these public health appointments originated from earlier health authority/local authority partnerships (for example, in Warwickshire and Walsall), some have direct PCT involvement, such as in Manchester, where the city's three PCTs and the city council have established a jointly funded public health unit (Hamer and Easton 2002).

Special project approaches

One traditional area of health improvement has been the development of special projects, either within or supported by primary care, that address wider determinants of inequalities in health. One example has been the development of welfare advice in general practice, with the support of citizen advice bureaux sessions in practices. These have been shown to improve the health status of patients (Abbott and Hobby 2000) and also encourage new clients, particularly those with a disability (Coppel *et al.* 1999). The use of advice workers in general practice has also shown benefits for families with young children, with positive benefits for maternal and child health (Reading *et al.* 2002).

The first two Tracker Surveys (Wilkin *et al.* 1999, 2001) found little evidence of community health initiatives and recent research on public involvement in primary care suggests that this activity was still a low priority for PCGs and PCTs (Harrison *et al.* 2002). In contrast, the most recent Tracker Survey did register an increase in the number of community development initiatives supported by PCTs (Gillam and Smith 2002). Heller (2002) also found that PCT representatives indicated that community initiatives were one of the main areas for developing public health work. Many PCG/Ts are also contributing resources to non-NHS initiatives, especially in the areas of community development, supporting family carers and accident prevention (Gillam and Smith 2002). However, while the majority did fund more than one such activity, the sums involved were fairly small and seldom exceeded £50,000 for any single project. Interestingly, where such developments are taking place, it is within areas where there are health action zones (Harrison *et al.* 2002). In the UK Public Health Association research we have also found the role of health action zones to be crucial in developing community-based work, although in our case study site there have been difficulties in transferring such activity into the new PCTs. This finding is reflected in the research on health improvement in London PCG/Ts (Abbott *et al.* 2001). This suggests that support for one-off projects, particularly those in the community, might not be as widespread or central to PCG/T approaches to public health as more mainstream NHS activity.

Organizational approaches of primary care trusts

Primary care trusts and their constituent parts are significant local agencies with large budgets. Clearly, they will have an effect on the health of their immediate employees. They can also make an important impact on their local communities through a range of human resource, purchasing, environmental and other organizational activities (Coote 2002). There is little evidence about activities such as these within the NHS as a whole, although policies using such approaches to maximize the benefit to, and well-being of, local communities have been used within local authorities. Nevertheless, some PCG/Ts have undertaken some schemes, including initiatives to employ and train local people in areas of high unemployment, paying attention to environmental improvements to premises, placing orders for consumables with local firms and so on.

The PCG/Ts can also act as good employers in the way they treat their staff. The review of NHS actions to tackle variations in health undertaken by the NHS Centre for Reviews and Dissemination (1985) recommended that NHS organizations should act as responsible employers in ways that promote good health. Although there has been some discussion about such approaches in informal settings and on public health electronic discussion lists, there is no current evidence to suggest that such approaches are being undertaken. This is an area that would be worthy of further research.

Primary care trusts and their communities

Primary care trusts are responsible for developing their own strategies for addressing local public health and including local communities. Some may have a history of joint working with other organizations to meet community needs; however, many more do not (Taylor *et al.* 1998; Hudson *et al.* 1999; Abbott *et al.* 2001). Involving the community in local public health issues within the context of developing local partnerships may be difficult and time-consuming. The government does not appear to want to be prescriptive about how the public is involved in public health activity, although there are more detailed guidelines and structures relating to public involvement in health care services (see Chapter 11). The key issue here seems to be that PCTs need to develop a clearer understanding of public health and how to engage local people (Gillam *et al.* 2001). This will take time, as will the subsequent development work.

The plans of PCTs for local action in public health need to demonstrate that the public has been involved in the development of these plans – especially health improvement and modernization plans – and that these plans are sensitive to local needs as well as meeting government targets (Department of Health 2002a). However, policy documents offer little guidance about how this can be achieved or about how primary care might fulfil its role as, for example, one of the partners in health action zone activity. In addition, the rhetoric in primary care organizations' plans about involving the community may not be reflected in actions. To date, PCG/Ts have not found it easy to address this aspect of public involvement (Wilkin *et al.* 1999; Anderson and Florin 2000). When they do attempt to involve the public, it is from a consumerist rather than a participative perspective; for example, patients giving feedback on existing services rather than being involved in a wider dialogue on health issues (Lupton *et al.* 1998; Taylor *et al.* 1998).

The public health activity of PCTs may be located in the community but primary care professionals do not necessarily engage with the community about public health issues or about the relevance of their activities to the community's priorities (Taylor *et al.* 1998). Generally, the organizational structures and cultures of primary care organizations reflect the predominant medical model, and this inhibits the development of community perspectives on health (Taylor *et al.* 1998). Therefore, professionals may confine their public health activity to a strictly medical agenda. Others, however, may go beyond their formal role to engage with the community on wider public health issues (Taylor *et al.* 1998; Wilkin *et al.* 1999; Anderson and Florin 2000; Abbott *et al.* 2001; Gillam and Smith 2002). This suggests that some PCTs may not formally sanction some forms of public health activity in the community. The findings of Taylor *et al.* (1998) suggest that engaging with the community about local public health issues means, among other things, addressing inequalities in the roles and relationships between professionals and with community members. Several factors may make this difficult. In the past, communities have not had a statutory right of access to processes that would allow them to influence decisions about health. The current changes in primary care have yet to identify clear processes and mechanisms for such involvement and recent guidance on patient and public involvement makes little reference to public health issues, as the new Patient Forums (see Chapter 11) are focused more on service delivery issues (Department of Health 2002b). Professionals may not engage with the public about the concerns of the community, may not agree with their concerns, or may not consider communication with the public on these matters even to be part of their role.

Conclusions: primary care trusts and public health – dependable, successful?

Most PCG/Ts feel they need more public health support and better information to discharge their health improvement responsibilities effectively. In a review of PCTs for the Health Development Agency, it was found that information is the most important aspect of the public health function in the PCT (Heller 2002), the emphasis being on information for preventive measures (immunization, screening), health needs assessment, evidence-based practice and guiding informed decision-making to improve health. Here the focus is on interventions to individuals, which suggests that respondents were not thinking about wider approaches to public health. In fact, PCT staff appear to feel that the barriers for tackling the wider determinants of health are enormous and have identified substantive training needs (Heller 2002; Petchey 2002).

Studies have also consistently identified the impact of organizational change on the ability to develop wider functions, such as partnership working (Hudson *et al.* 1999; Coleman and Glendinning 2002) and developing public health activity (Abbott *et al.* 2001; Gillam *et al.* 2001). This has also been a key factor in the UK Public Health Association research, where the transition to PCTs and new network and partnership arrangements were found to have cut across long-standing relationships; focused attention on organizational development; and placed the NHS agenda more centrally in their work, thereby often marginalizing other, more locally driven agendas. In addition, studies have also found that the move to PCT status has shifted their focus of attention from looking 'inwards and downwards' to their local communities (responding to local needs and demands) to looking 'outwards and upwards' (being more focused on national targets, priorities and central government directives) (Abbott *et al.* 2001; Heller 2002). The UK Public Health Association research is also finding that PCG/Ts are shifting their focus in this way.

However, this has meant that there has been discussion and activity in relation to the national service frameworks. UK Public Health Association fieldwork has found that practices and PCTs are prioritizing public health work with older people, people with mental health problems and so on, although this is not uniform across all practices. However, there is some reason to expect that the inclusion of health inequality targets in the recent *Improvement, Expansion and Reform: The Next 3 Years. Priorities and Planning Framework 2003–2006* (Department of Health 2002c) will mean that PCTs are likely to place a greater emphasis on this area of work. Nevertheless, despite the evidence that more PCTs are developing partnership work, there are still grounds for concern as to the extent to which this will develop beyond organizational arrangements such as participating in local strategic partnerships.

The emphasis on medical knowledge, reactive approaches to health and the dominance of medical culture and organization within the NHS, particularly primary care, suggests that PCTs may find it difficult to work collaboratively with either professional partners or with the public on wider public health issues (Taylor *et al.* 1998). Such a focus may also lead to a poor understanding of public health beyond the confines of the medical model. Yet most survey work with PCG/Ts, and the fieldwork currently being undertaken for the UK Public Health Association Study, have found that staff in PCG/Ts have tremendous optimism about the development of public health within this new organizational framework. This reflects findings in relation to partnership working (Hudson *et al.* 1999). Given the complex organizational change that is currently occurring within PCTs and the shift towards new areas of activity such as public health, it is perhaps too soon to provide an assessment of success or even dependability.

References

Abbott, S. and Hobby, L. (2000) Welfare benefits advice in primary care: evidence of improvements in health, *Public Health*, 114(5): 324–7.

Abbott, S., Florin, D., Fulop, N. and Gillam, S. (2001) *Primary Care Groups and Trusts: Improving Health*. London: King's Fund.

Anderson, W. and Florin, D. (2000) *Involving the Public – One of Many Priorities*. London: King's Fund.

Ashenden, R., Silagy, C. and Weller, D. (1997) A systematic review of the effectiveness of promoting lifestyle change in general practice, *Family Practice*, 14(2): 160–75.

Baggott, R. (2000) *The Politics of Public Health*. Basingstoke: Macmillan.

Biles, A., Mornement, A. and Palmer, H. (2001) From the ballot box to the real world, *Regeneration and Renewal*, 8 June, pp. 14–15.

Braham, P. and Janes, L. (2002) *Social Differences and Divisions*. Oxford: Blackwell.

Burke, S., Meyrick, J. and Speller, V. (2001) *Public Health Skills Audit 2001*. London: HDA.

Butler, C.C., Pill, R. and Stott, N.C.H. (1998) Qualitative study of patients' perceptions of doctors' advice to quit smoking: implications for opportunistic health promotion, *British Medical Journal*, 316: 1878–81.

Carr-Hill, R. and Chalmers-Dixon, P. (2002) *A Review of Methods for Monitoring and Measuring Social Inequality, Deprivation and Health Inequality*. Web-based report, Centre for Health Economics, University of York (http://www.sepho.org.uk/HealthInequalities/carrhill/index.htm).

Chief Medical Officer (2001) *The Report of the Chief Medical Officer's Project to Strengthen the Public Health Function*. London: Department of Health.

Clamp, M. and Kendrick, D. (1998) A randomised controlled trial of general practitioner safety advice for families with children under 5 years, *British Medical Journal*, 316: 1576–9.

Coleman, A. and Glendinning, C. (2002) Partnerships, in D. Wilkin, A. Coleman, B. Dowling and K. Smith (eds) *The National Tracker Survey of Primary Care Groups and Trusts 2001/2002: Taking Responsibility?* Manchester: National Primary Care Research and Development Centre.

Coote, A. (2002) *Claiming the Health Divide*. London: King's Fund.

Coppel, D.H., Packham, C.J. and Varnam, M.A. (1999) Providing welfare rights in primary care, *Public Health*, 113(3): 131–5.

Department of the Environment, Transport and the Regions (2000) *Our Towns and Cities*. London: DETR.

Department of the Environment, Transport and the Regions (2001) *Local Strategic Partnerships: Government Guidance*. London: DETR.

Department of Health (1993) *Public Health Responsibilities of the NHS and Others (Abrams Committee Report)*. London: Department of Health.

Department of Health (2001a) *Shifting the Balance of Power in the NHS: Securing Delivery*. London: Department of Health.

Department of Health (2001b) *Tackling Health Inequalities: Consultation on a Plan for Delivery*. London: Department of Health.

Department of Health (2002a) *Shifting the Balance: Next Steps*. London: The Stationery Office.

Department of Health (2002b) *Patient and Public Involvement: The Future Picture*. London: Department of Health.

Department of Health (2002c) *Improvement, Expansion and Reform: The Next 3 Years. Priorities and Planning Framework 2003–2006*. London: Department of Health.

Department of Health and Social Security (1988) *Public Health in England: The Report of the Committee of Inquiry into the Future Development of the Public Health Function* (The Acheson Report). London: HMSO.

Faculty of Public Health Medicine and Health Development Agency (2001) *Statement on Managed Public Health Networks*. London: Faculty of Public Health Medicine and Health Development Agency.

Fitzpatrick, M. (2001) *The Tyranny of Health: Doctors and the Regulation of Lifestyle*. London: Routledge.

Gillam, S. and Smith, K. (2002) Health Improvement, in D. Wilkin, A. Coleman, B. Dowling and K. Smith (eds) *The National Tracker Survey of Primary Care Groups and Trusts 2001/2002: Taking Responsibility?* Manchester: National Primary Care Research and Development Centre.

Gillam, S., Abbott, S. and Banks-Smith, J. (2001) Can primary care groups and trusts improve health?, *British Medical Journal*, 323: 89–92.

Goddard, M. and Smith, P. (2001) Equity of access to health care services: theory and evidence from the UK, *Social Science and Medicine*, 53(9): 1149–62.

Hamer, L. and Easton, N. (2002) *Community Strategies and Health Improvement: A Review of Policy and Practice*. London: HDA.

Harrison, S., Milewa, T. and Dowswell, G. (2002) *Patient and Public Involvement in Primary Care Organisations*. Final Report to the Department of Health. Manchester: The University of Manchester.

Heller, D. (2002) *How can primary care trusts develop and implement their public health roles to help reduce health inequalities?* Paper to the HDA Seminar on Tackling Health Inequalities, London, June 2002.

Hudson, B., Callaghan, G., Exworthy, M. and Peckham, S. (1999) *Locality Partnerships: The Early PCG Experience*. Report to Northern and Yorkshire NHS Executive R&D.

Hulscher, M., Wensing, M., van der Weijden, T. and Grol, R. (2001) Interventions to implement prevention in primary care (Cochrane Review), in *The Cochrane Library*, Issue 1. Oxford: Update Software.

Lennox, A.S., Osman, L.M., Reiter, E. *et al.* (2001) Cost effectiveness of computer tailored and non-tailored smoking cessation letters in general practice: randomised controlled trial, *British Medical Journal*, 322(7299): 1396–1400.

Levenson, R. and Johnson, L. (2000) *Improving Health at the Local Level: The Role of Primary Care*. London: King's Fund.

Lewis, J. (1986) *What Price Community Medicine? The Philosophy, Practice and Politics of Public Health Since 1919*. Brighton: Wheatsheaf.

Lupton, C., Peckham, S. and Taylor, P. (1998) *Managing Public Involvement in Healthcare Purchasing*. Buckingham: Open University Press.

Macdonald, J. (1992) *Primary Health Care: Medicine in its Place*. London: Earthscan.

Meads, G., Killoran, A., Ashcroft, J. and Cornish, Y. (1999) *Mixing Oil and Water: How Can Primary Care Organisations Improve Health as Well as Deliver Effective Health Care?* London: Health Education Authority.

NHS Centre for Reviews and Dissemination (1995) *Review of the Research on the Effectiveness of Health Service Interventions to Reduce Variations in Health*. York: The University of York.

Peckham, S. and Godel, M. (2001) Primary care, communities and public health, *Health Matters*, 44: 18.

Peckham, S. and Exworthy, M. (2002) *Primary Care in the UK: Policy, Organisation and Management*. Basingstoke: Palgrave Macmillan.

Petchey, R. (2002) *PCTs and public health: learning from research*. Paper presented at Great Expectations or Hard Times? Primary Care Trusts and Public Health Conference, London, 17 June.

Popay, J. (2001) *Evidence to House of Commons Select Committee on Health*. London: The Stationery Office.

Pratt, J. (1995) *Practitioners and Practices: A Conflict of Values?* Oxford: Radcliffe Medical Press.

Reading, R., Steel, S. and Reynolds, S. (2002) Citizens advice in primary care for families with young children, *Child Care Health Development*, 28(1): 39–45.

Scott, T. (2002) *Report of the First Meeting of the Joint NHS Leadership Centre and Faculty of Public Health Medicine, Public Health Leadership Thinking and Planning Group*, NHS Leadership Centre, Oxford, 16–17 May.

Secretary of State for Health (1997) *The New NHS: Modern, Dependable*. London: The Stationery Office.

Secretary of State for Health (1998) *Our Healthier Nation*. London: The Stationery Office.

Secretary of State for Health (1999) *Saving lives: Our Healthier Nation*. London: The Stationery Office.

Secretary of State for Health (2000) *The NHS Plan: A Plan for Investment, a Plan for Reform*. London: The Stationery Office.

Smeeth, L. and Heath, I. (1999) Tackling health inequalities in primary care, *British Medical Journal*, 318: 1020–1.

Starfield, B. (1998) *Primary Care: Balancing Health Needs, Services and Technology*. New York: Oxford University Press.

Taylor, P., Peckham, S. and Turton, P. (1998) *A Public Health Model of Primary Care: From Concept to Reality*. Birmingham: Public Health Alliance.

Tudor-Hart, J. (1988) *A New Kind of Doctor*. London: Merlin Press.

Wilkin, D., Gillam, S. and Leese, B. (eds) (2000) *The National Tracker Survey of Primary Care Groups and Trusts: Progress and Challenges 1999/2000*. Manchester: National Primary Care Research and Development Centre.

Wilkin, D., Gillam, S. and Coleman, A. (eds) (2001) *The National Tracker Survey of Primary Care Groups and Trusts 2000/2001: Modernising the NHS?* Manchester: The University of Manchester.

Wilkin, D., Coleman, A., Dowling, B. and Smith, K. (eds) (2002) *The National Tracker Survey of Primary Care Groups and Trusts 2001/2002: Taking Responsibility?* Manchester: The University of Manchester.

Wilkinson, R.G. (1996) *Unhealthy Societies*. London: Routledge

Wirrmann, E. (2002) *Public health activity in general practice: establishing a basis for strengthening the public health function in primary care*. Paper presented at the British Sociological Association Medical Sociology Group Conference, York, September 2002.

Woodhead, D., Jochelson, K. and Tennant, R. (2002) *Public Health in the Balance: Getting it Right for London*. London: King's Fund.

11 Public involvement and democratic accountability in primary care organizations

Timothy Milewa, Stephen Harrison and George Dowswell

Introduction

The National Health Service (NHS) retains a symbolic and material, if often strained, role as the keystone of collective welfare provision in the UK. But a post-war tradition of centralized administrative control and deference to a powerful medical profession have remained largely unchallenged, despite sustained attempts to increase the influence of those in whose name the service was founded — citizens and patients. Since the early 1990s, however, the notion of public and patient involvement has attracted a considerable amount of political exhortation and guidance, especially since 1997 and especially in relation to primary health care.

This chapter begins with a brief overview of the history of democracy and accountability in the NHS. It then draws upon research conducted between 1999 and 2001 to address four issues related to public and patient involvement in the planning of primary health care by the principal organizations at this level of the NHS, primary care groups (PCGs) and primary care trusts (PCTs). First, we use the results from a national survey to gauge the extent to which involvement features on organizational agendas and is being realized through particular initiatives at a local level. Second, we compare professional and lay views on the criteria by which the impact of involvement could and should be measured. Third, we focus upon the initial thoughts of these stakeholders on the success or failure of initiatives with which they are acquainted. Finally, we move from a focus on the relationship between primary care groups and trusts (PCG/Ts) and local populations to a consideration of how public and patient involvement may influence relationships between key actor-groups within these organizations. The focus here is upon the relationship between the new, increasingly prominent, managerial strata charged with running PCTs and the old, traditionally powerful general practitioners (GPs) upon whom the organizations are based. In conclusion, we consider the implications of our findings for future approaches to public and patient involvement in primary care organizations.

Democracy, accountability and health care planning in context

Concerns about the influence wielded by citizens and patients over decision-making within the NHS are hardly new. Indeed, plans in the 1940s initially envisaged governance of the new health service by joint boards of existing local government authorities (Foot 1973). However, the 1945 Labour government subsequently gave only community and ambulance services to the latter, leaving the two remaining elements of the tripartite NHS, the hospitals and family (medical, dental, pharmaceutical and optical) practitioners, to be governed by appointed bodies. The National Health Service Act 1946 emphasized the central political direction of the service; appointed management bodies were 'to administer the service consistent with the directives of the minister and relevant regulations' (Webster 1988: 95). At the same time, this arrangement distanced the administrative (rather than managerial) function from both local electoral politics and any nascent notions of citizen self-advocacy, leaving the local scene balanced between central appointees and representatives of the professions. Thus, in the field of primary health care the composition of executive councils (responsible for holding the contracts of the self-employed family practitioners of medicine, dentistry and pharmacy) was finely balanced between professional representatives (seven from the local medical committee, three from the local dental committee and two from the local pharmaceutical committee) and government appointees (five plus the chair appointed by the minister, eight by the relevant local government health authorities) (Webster 1988). Indeed, despite some official discussion in the mid-1950s, the possibility of a greater role for local government was not seriously considered again until the latter part of the 1960s, when two proposals that the NHS should be wholly governed by the new local government authorities were floated (Royal Commission 1969; Department of Health and Social Security 1970). However, the major reorganization of the NHS in 1974 did not reflect this line of thought. Instead, the focus was upon the partial unification of the three parts of the tripartite structure. Appointed regional health authorities and area health authorities were to be responsible for hospital and community services, the latter therefore being lost by local authorities except for the right to appoint to a few places on the new authorities. Executive councils would become family practitioner committees.

The absence of appointees with an explicit remit to represent the interests of ordinary people in the health service did, however, inform the creation in 1974 of community health councils to represent the interests of the public in the NHS within each health district. Half of the membership was nominated by local government authorities, a third by voluntary organizations and the remaining sixth by regional health authorities (Levitt and Wall 1984). The idea of local elected control over the NHS did not disappear entirely, but the Royal Commission on the NHS established by the Labour government in 1976 (reporting in 1979) rejected the notion of elected single-purpose health authorities (Royal Commission 1979) and, in relation to primary care, the notion of appointment according to sectional interests continued. Eleven members of each family practitioner committee were to be nominated by the health authority, four by the local authority, eight by the local medical committee, three by the local dental committee, and two each by the local optical and pharmaceutical committees (Levitt and Wall 1984). Moreover, after the abolition of area health authorities in 1982, when family practitioner committees were later restyled as family health services authorities, they gained independence from other local health governance arrangements and became responsible directly to the Department of Health. Moreover, unlike other authorities, family practitioner committees were not required to hold public meetings until 1983 (Allsop and May 1986).

However, the creation of a managerial (as opposed to administrative) function in the 1980s and attempts in the early 1990s to introduce some 'market discipline' to the health service implied at least a rhetorical concern for the responsiveness of GPs to patients. The creation in 1991 of a quasi-market in the NHS sought to enhance flexibility and service responsiveness by separating the purchasing or planning role from that of service provision. Health authorities, the purchasers, were thus exhorted for most of the 1990s to actively gauge the views and preferences of their local populations (Milewa *et al.* 1998), even though their former local authority membership had been abandoned in favour of a structure more like that of a commercial board of directors. This period also saw an attempt to turn GPs into purchasers through the medium of fundholding status, under which practices could volunteer to assume budgetary control over aspects of staffing, some hospital services and drug prescribing. Fundholding, it seems to have been assumed, would somehow empower patients, though the only obvious mechanism was that it became slightly easier for patients to change GPs and for patients to obtain information about their GP's services. The little evidence that is available on this aspect of fundholding suggests that GPs found it difficult to believe in the value of being responsive to patients or the public collectively, or to commit themselves to formal consultative mechanisms (Dixon *et al.* 1998; Brown 2000).

New labour and involvement

In formal terms at least, the Labour governments of 1997 and 2001 considerably intensified the policy focus on patient and public involvement, especially in primary care. The creation in 1999 of 481 PCGs, based on local groups of general practices and other primary care professionals, was therefore accompanied by a requirement that they develop mechanisms for the early, systematic and continuous involvement of users and the public (Department of Health 1998a). This exhortation continued as PCGs moved from the status of non-statutory committees of health authorities to that of quasi-autonomous statutory organizations, PCTs. Indeed, at least half the members of the boards of PCTs would, it was decided, be lay (rather than professional) in terms of their background. But this stipulation should be treated with some caution because the term 'lay', in this context, can include retired health care professionals and those based in areas outside the localities administered by a particular PCT; in short, some lay members were doctors. A wealth of official policy and guidance documents about patient and public involvement was published, including *Patient and Public Involvement in the New NHS* (Department of Health 1999), parts of *The NHS Plan* (Secretary of State for Health 2000), *Involving Patients and the Public in Health Care* (Department of Health 2001a) and *Patient Representation in the New NHS* (Department of Health 2001b). Concrete institutional reform was, however, preceded by a period of debate, indecision and, in the case of plans to abolish community health councils, conflict between 1999 and 2002.

There followed a considerable amount of organizational change, four strands of which, by the summer of 2002, were becoming clear (Transition Advisory Board for Patient and Public Involvement in Health 2002). In placing the findings reported in this chapter within context, these developments are perhaps most interesting for what they tell us about particular official understandings of what constitutes involvement and who it is that the government expects to become involved.

Patients' forums

At the most local level, every PCT is required to constitute a patients' forum, drawn largely from among local patients and residents. These bodies appear to reflect a focus upon public/citizen consultation, particularly with regard to prospective decisions about services. The forums thus inform, but do not directly shape or steer, professional decisions (a passive rather than participatory role for local people). In broad terms, the forums will monitor and review the services commissioned or provided by PCTs from the perspective of the patient; actively gauge the views and experiences of patients; and present such information to PCTs and other local decision-makers. This role will be facilitated in part by the right of forums to inspect premises in which NHS care is provided. The forums will also be expected to monitor the extent to which local NHS bodies are meeting their statutory obligation to consult and involve the public. Indeed, the forums are also expected to promote the involvement of local people in consultations and decisions that affect health, a pro-active role paralleled by their power to either provide or commission independent schemes for complaint advocacy. Finally, in raising particular issues, each forum will be able to make use of representation on PCT boards through a non-executive director and, perhaps more significantly, to refer issues to external bodies and the media as they deem appropriate.

Patient advice and liaison services

Each PCT will also develop a patient advice and liaison service (PALS). These bodies will have several functions but overall will act as conduits for complaints and sources of information for individuals. Once again, the focus is not upon involving local citizens or patients in making decisions about services (although trends in complaints and requests for information might conceivably be used in the development of services). Instead, these bodies will seek, if possible, to resolve patient concerns and complaints at an early stage. The service will also provide a single point for information and advice to patients, carers and families, and serve as the entry point to other avenues of advocacy and complaint. In addition, the patient advice and liaison service will monitor trends and highlight deficiencies in local health care services as part of an 'early warning' process; concerns will be expressed in formal reports for action to PCTs, as well as through less formal feedback. These recommendations, and the specific responses of PCTs, will feature in annual prospectuses for patients that the PCTs will be obliged to produce and each patient advice and liaison service will provide anonymous reports to the relevant patients' forum to enhance responsiveness in the NHS.

Overview and scrutiny committees

Overview and scrutiny committees, already in existence to oversee local authority functions, constitute a third type of involvement – a quasi-electoral form. Constituted by local authorities that are run by elected members, the committees will have four main roles in relation to local NHS activities. First, subject to consultation on regulations and guidance, all local NHS bodies will have a duty to provide information about their activities and services to the new committees and NHS chief executives may be required to attend relevant meetings to answer questions. Second, the committees will be able to make recommendations to NHS bodies that, in the event of disagreement, will be required to provide reasons for the rejection of these ideas. Third, there will be a specific NHS duty to consult the local overview and scrutiny committee on proposed major changes in local health services. Finally, if a committee disagrees with a proposed change (or is of the opinion that there has been inadequate local consultation or involvement in reaching a decision about local health services), it will be able to refer the matter to the Secretary of State for Health.

Commission for patient and public involvement in health

The fourth innovation appears to be a fairly novel aspect of involvement, that of regulatory governance. At a national level – far removed from the minutiae of local health services and associated conflicts – the Commission for Patient and Public Involvement in Health (CPPIH) is charged with four main activities. First, the commission will report to the Secretary of State for Health on the overall performance of general arrangements for public and patient involvement in the NHS and offer advice as appropriate. Second, it will be able to offer advice and reports to other relevant bodies, such as the Commission for Health Improvement, on public and patient involvement and issues of patient welfare that are not being addressed through other means. Third, more specifically, it will monitor and advise on the performance of patients' forums and bodies responsible for supporting independent complaints and advocacy, including setting appropriate standards. Fourthly, the commission will conduct national reviews of services from the perspective of patients (perhaps drawing on data collected by patients' forums). Such reviews may inform recommendations to the Secretary of State for Health and to any other individuals or organizations deemed appropriate.

These new mechanisms (consultation with local publics; a channel for individual complaints/requests for information; quasi-electoral representation of local communities; and a national policing role with regard to involvement) overlook a fifth – pre-existing and ongoing – type of involvement. This centres on the role of patients, users and citizen groups as autonomous stakeholders or partners in discussions surrounding local health services, a qualitatively different notion to the idea of top-down consultation, individual grievance procedures or representation by third parties (Milewa *et al.* 2002a). Accordingly in the study reported in this chapter, we were concerned to draw a very basic distinction between official stakeholders (in this case, personnel formally connected to PCG/Ts) and other stakeholders (based upon autonomous service user, pressure or community groups). We sought, among other topics, to examine some of the issues that might differentiate the views of different stakeholders about the impact of public and patient involvement and to consider the early implications of involvement for relationships between stakeholders within PCG/Ts. We address four specific questions in this chapter:

- To what extent are PCG/Ts addressing involvement through specific attempts to engage local people?
- Do stakeholders within PCG/Ts have similar ideas to user/voluntary/ community sector stakeholders about the criteria against which the impact of involvement can be gauged?
- Do stakeholders within PCG/Ts have similar ideas to user/voluntary/ community sector stakeholders about any changes attributable to early initiatives in public and patient involvement?
- Does public and patient involvement influence the relationship between PCT managers and a third group of stakeholders, GPs, in any way?

Method

In addressing these questions, the research employed four means of data collection:

- Semi-structured telephone interviews were conducted between November 1999 and March 2000 with spokespersons of PCG/Ts in a target random sample of half the groups outside London ($n = 208$). After piloting, interviews were conducted with 167 informants (a response rate of just over 80 per cent)
- Semi-structured face-to-face interviews were conducted with a purposive snowball sample of 68 informants from three health authority districts between November 2000 and May 2001. Of this sample, 32 individuals were attached to eleven PCG/Ts in the three districts; 29 were drawn from local voluntary, community or residents' organizations; and the remaining seven from other statutory bodies, such as health authorities, local authorities and NHS community mental health trusts.
- A second round of semi-structured face-to-face interviews was conducted between June and September 2001 with 42 informants in the district within which PCTs (as opposed to PCGs) had been established the longest (the pseudonymous Redtown). This time we interviewed 42 informants, of whom 15 were attached to the four PCTs in the district, 18 were drawn from the community and voluntary sectors and another nine from the non-PCT statutory sector.
- Telephone interviews were carried out with spokespersons nominated by a random 20 per cent sample of general practices in Redtown ($n = 20$) in September 2001.

Public and patient involvement: a national picture and local focus

Over 85 per cent of respondents to the national survey indicated that their PCG/Ts either had or were in the process of formulating a strategy or action plan with regard to public and patient involvement. More than 98 per cent of PCG/Ts could cite particular initiatives for involving the public and patients that had been adopted. Those cited most frequently included visits by PCG/T members to meetings of patient, voluntary or advocacy groups; liaison with locality groups or forums (based variously on service users, local residents, health and social care professionals and the voluntary sector); newsletters; and membership of existing networks composed of statutory and voluntary sector organizations.

Nearly 44 per cent of the 167 PCG/Ts reported at least one initiative oriented specifically to marginalized groups who, in the view of informants, might be overlooked without a particular effort by the PCG/Ts to engage them in dialogue. More than 26 per cent of these initiatives were focused upon minority ethnic communities. A further 16 per cent of the activities were oriented towards older people and similar proportions were aimed at people with mental health problems and deprived populations (such as those on depressed housing estates). A small proportion of activities (less than 8 per cent) were geared towards those with physical impairments, while people with learning disabilities were targeted by under 5 per cent of the activities.

When informants were asked if involvement activities had resulted in demonstrable changes to PCG/T policies or plans, just over 29 per cent cited examples in sufficient detail to be recorded. Among these 50 specific changes, the largest proportion (28 per cent) centred on provision of additional services (such as physiotherapy, or advice to teenagers on contraception and sexual health). Another 24 per cent of changes were to plans for the location or reconfiguration of services, in particular the location of general practices and pharmacies. Revisions to health improvement plans accounted for 16 per cent of recorded changes, while significant amendments to other documents amounted to 18 per cent of such changes. A further 10 per cent of changes centred on procedural issues, such as the acoustics and seating arrangements for meetings open to the public (Milewa *et al.* 2002b).

Involvement in local context

The involvement activities reported in the national survey tended to be echoed in the three districts that were investigated more closely. These activities fell into two broad categories: first, the use of existing 'community development' conduits beyond the PCG/Ts; second, reliance upon internally instigated mechanisms. If, for example, we focus on the four PCTs in the pseudonymous district of Redtown, the external conduits that were utilized included attendance at meetings of voluntary and community groups. Personnel from one PCT, for example, attended a community group's meeting to discuss the content of planned personal medical services contracts with general practices in the locality, while informants from another PCT reported a visit to a district-wide group for older users of health and social services. All four PCTs sent representatives to the local authority's neighbourhood forums or area panels, although there were mixed feelings among informants about the utility of these. There also appeared to have been a clear movement among the PCTs towards representation on voluntary or quasi-voluntary organizations. For example, one PCT was represented on a multi-sector community involvement group of relatively long-standing in the district, while the chairperson of another PCT sat on the management committee of a carers' organization.

The internally instigated mechanisms and conduits deployed by the four PCTs in Redtown included joint funding of a college-based course designed to enhance the advocacy and self-advocacy skills of local individuals and groups in the voluntary and community sector. Informants from all four PCTs mentioned seminars or workshops on particular issues. These included a networking event on community safety, a meeting of people involved in Health Action Zone-funded projects and a special 'health day' that involved meetings with a range of community leaders. All PCTs also mentioned producing newsletters and, although several informants mentioned websites, only one indicated that their website would allow for some degree of interactivity on the part of users (primarily for searching for very specific information and contacting particular functions within the PCT). Only one PCT mentioned the use of formal health forums or panels, one in each of the trust's three localities, and only two of the four PCTs reported the use of formally constituted patient reference groups. In the case of one of Redtown's PCTs, for example, such groups were established in relation to coronary heart disease/angina, cancer and mental health. Other strategies employed by the PCTs included public or patient representation on subcommittees or working groups, such as lay representation on a clinical governance subgroup.

How did different stakeholders measure the impact of involvement?

Thoughts on how the impact of involvement might be gauged reflected an apparent division between stakeholders within PCG/Ts (hereafter 'PCT informants') and those from voluntary, community and other statutory organizations (hereafter 'non-PCT informants'). First, non-PCT informants placed considerably more emphasis than PCT stakeholders upon demonstrable changes in services or improvements in health; this was particularly the case in the pseudonymous districts of Redtown and Bluetown. A community health council spokesperson in Redtown said:

> I referred earlier to the gap between expectations and actual services on the ground. And I would want to be seeing a closing of that gap, that there was more congruence between people's expectations and the service that they actually receive – that would be a measure of success.

Non-PCT informants were also more inclined to cite specific process indicators, such as the participation of senior PCT personnel or the size of budgets devoted to involvement activities:

> One of our other priority actions is to develop indicators that demonstrate the effectiveness or not of involvement within the PCT . . . We're hoping that we'll be able to use some of the King's Fund stuff as well . . . Early indicators would be level of core budget committed – that indicates a level of commitment to the work. Key PCT personnel having lead functions and roles – that's another indicator.

PCT informants, on the other hand, attached considerably greater importance than their non-PCT counterparts to more general feedback from the public and patients, either directly or through various systems of internal review. Some PCT informants, but no non-PCT informants, also saw a greater awareness of the PCG/Ts and their role as indicative of the success of involvement initiatives. The lay member of a Bluetown PCG board spoke of the use of feedback and a community involvement worker in another of the city's groups commented on the importance of raised public awareness about the new organizations:

> The success would be if you develop services that are well received and the feedback is positive. You can measure it in terms of people attending meetings – people have had their say as we go through the [consultation process prior to PCT status]; people write down in minutes all the questions answered.

> So ten people who have become smoking cessation advisers didn't know anything about the PCG – but now they've been in the building, they know the people and it makes [the PCG] more accessible. So they say, 'Oh yeah, I can see what they're doing'.

Were these differences between the views of PCT and non-PCT informants, about the criteria by which involvement's impact should be judged, echoed by perceptions of actual change; and, if so, could this be attributed to public and patient involvement at a local level?

Perceptions of the impact of involvement

Responses here clustered around three themes. First, the non-PCT informants in all three districts were considerably more inclined than PCT interviewees to argue that no demonstrable changes could yet be linked to involvement activities on the part of PCG/Ts. This was not so much cynicism as a general awareness of the new organizations' relative youth:

> It's much too early days yet, it really is early days. [The PCT] have been far too concerned with getting the structures right I think, and not looking at the actual delivery side of things.

Non-PCTinformantswerealsolessinclinedthanPCTstakeholderstoattribute specific changes in service delivery or service procedures to public and patient involvement. Indeed, in the pseudonymous district of Greentown, PCT informants cited a handful of such changes, but non-PCT informants could not provide any examples of changes in service delivery or procedures that they could link to public or patient input. Examples of change cited by PCT informants in Greentown included evening opening by a general practice and customer care training for general practice receptionists. Instances of change as a result of involvement cited by PCT informants in Redtown included the development of rehabilitation and palliative care services and changed opening and appointment systems in a general practice. Claimed changes in Bluetown included the relocation of physiotherapy services and enhanced telephone access to health care facilities.

However, similar proportions of both PCT and non-PCT informants claimed that substantive changes to organizational agendas or action plans (rather than specific changes on the ground) had arisen as a result of involvement. Issues mentioned included local transport and access to health services in Redtown, the signposting of services within and between particular care settings, and the development of standards for local nursing homes. The type of dialogues that led to such agenda changes was illustrated by the lay member of a PCG board in Bluetown in relation to mental health:

> City councillors made us aware of mental health; people we spoke to in the street, a few groups I spoke to in the early days, all talked about mental health and drug problems. And of course I fed that back and it's become a more active interest of the PCG because it was acknowledged that not just we (as board members, GPs and community staff) but that the public were talking about it as well.

Finally, as a number of informants noted, PCG/Ts were still young organizations. We were therefore also interested in their views on the future impact
of public and patient involvement. Informants were asked whether it would be
possible, at some future date, to link involvement activities to specific changes.
The PCT informants tended to be considerably more optimistic in this respect
than non-PCT interviewees. The Bluetown PCG board's lay member reflected
the positive line of thought, but a voluntary sector informant in the same
district was more pessimistic:

> On the grand scheme of things, at primary care level, I think that you
> will see more user-friendly GPs, more localized services – a return
> perhaps to that perspective where GPs actually treat people rather
> than writing letters of referral . . . But it's only going back to what was
> around in the 1950s, not that I was around.

> Health has always been very aloof, health has always known what's
> best – nothing's changed. And it seems to me that nothing is going to
> change – they know everything. Consultation, they don't know what
> it actually means.

As this last observation implies, the policy and practice of involvement can be
framed in terms other than the relationship between health care planners and
the public and patients whose interests they supposedly serve. How, for
instance, did the issue of involvement impact upon the relationship between
PCT managers and GPs?

Doctors, managers and involvement

In looking at the relationship between doctors, managers and the issue of
public and patient involvement, we focused on the district Redtown, within
which PCTs had been established the longest. The four PCTs in Redtown, like
all others, are premised on the notion of federations of GPs; but PCTs also have
a clear management structure in place. Strategic vision and corporate accountability rest with chief executives, the board and functional directors, while
members of the primary health care professions sit on professional executive
committees within the PCT. These arrangements do not challenge directly the
influence of GPs and other health care professionals but do represent a further
accentuation of the managerial ethos that took hold in the NHS in the 1980s
and 1990s, a trend made explicit with an official emphasis on the need for
systems and processes of corporate governance that echo those in the private
sector. Indeed, three of the PCTs indicated that requirements relating to
obtaining patient views or involving service users would routinely form part of

personal medical services (PMS) contracts with general practices. A PCT chief executive explained:

> We've got eleven out of the thirteen practices in PMS . . . What we've actually said is that they have to do a number of things – we've given them a menu. So they have to do two or three out of six things. One of them is set up, this year, their own patient forum. There are other things involving patient involvement.

There was little evidence of hostility or opposition on the part of GPs but, anecdotally, mention was made of weariness and a degree of suspicion on the part of doctors with regard to the involvement agenda. The chair of another PCT explained:

> We had the joint meeting of the professional executive committee and the board which looked at public involvement, which got quite heated. It was the doctors who felt that they were being asked to do one too many a thing and being asked in a manner that felt a bit confrontational.

However, as some other informants observed, the idea of patient involvement at a general practice level is hardly new. So, despite the reservations of some GPs, to what extent were the PCTs building upon existing, rather than instigating new, forms of involvement at a practice level? Results from a telephone survey of a random sample of twenty general practices (20 per cent) in Redtown were mixed. Half the informants (mainly practice managers, who had been given advance notice of the questions) were aware of activities or debate within the PCT about patient and public involvement, but the same proportion indicated that none of their GPs were actively interested in public and patient involvement. A further six respondents indicated that at least one doctor in their practice was strongly supportive of such involvement and two informants reported that at least one of their GPs was strongly against the idea of involvement. Public and patient involvement was apparently not seen as a direct or urgent threat to the power and autonomy of GPs, but instead represented one strand of guidance among many requirements of PCTs. However, the government has argued that the price of professional autonomy for doctors is that they must be 'openly accountable for the standards they set and the way these are enforced' and that 'these standards must take account of legitimate public expectations and the realities of service delivery locally' (Department of Health 1998b: 46). It may therefore become the case that corporate governance, clinical governance and patient and public involvement become increasingly inseparable elements of PCT organizational agendas.

Conclusions

Our national survey indicated that public and patient involvement is now on the agenda of most PCG/Ts and our qualitative research in three districts confirmed that significant efforts were often being made to develop strategies and mechanisms for involvement. However, we also saw significant differences between PCT and non-PCT informants in the criteria that each thought should be used to gauge the impact of involvement and a similar difference of views on the actual changes attributable to such involvement; informants from the voluntary and community sector tended to be more sceptical. Nevertheless, the study also found some tentative evidence to suggest that the issue of patient and public involvement is increasingly being used as a medium in the relationship between PCTs (and perhaps the government) and GPs. Taking the findings as a whole, is it possible to draw any inferences about the role of PCTs in taking forward the issue of involvement as part of the so-called 'modernization' of the NHS?

First, the fieldwork reported here was conducted at a time of considerable change and innovation in the structures concerned with public and patient involvement in primary care planning and development. As we hinted at the start of this chapter, new arrangements such as patients' forums represent particular types of involvement and could actually be seen to reflect a trend towards the fragmentation and containment of public and patient views. Local people have been cast as 'the consulted' (patients' forums), as individuals with a complaint or a need for specific information (patient advice and liaison services), as an electoral constituency (overview and scrutiny committees) and as the governed (Commission for Patient and Public Involvement in Health). But participatory involvement – founded on the notion of autonomous user, voluntary or community stakeholders who choose how and when to engage with service planners – is at best regarded as an implicit form of engagement. This implicit recognition may not be problematic in itself. However, any stakeholders that operate beyond these official and apparently comprehensive channels of dialogue run the risk of having their legitimacy or suitability to be representatives questioned. So, paradoxically, the apparent breadth of new formal conduits of engagement may actually constrict the extent to which local service users and citizens are able, as legitimate stakeholders or partners in the planning process, to challenge professional decisions. Primary care trusts will thus play a central role in determining not only what constitutes involvement but in demarcating those who are regarded as legitimate participants in this respect.

Secondly, the different emphases placed by non-PCT and PCT stakeholders on the impact of involvement raises the question of whether there will continue to be a supply of people willing to be involved. If lay participants differ from professionals in their perceptions of the impact of involvement (and, as discussed above, in relation to what constitutes involvement), is there a long-term future for significant patient and public involvement? It would be premature to attempt an answer to this question, but it is worth noting that the research reported here is broadly consistent with that of other contemporary studies (Anderson and Florin 2000; Bond et al. 2001; North and Peckham 2001; Alborz et al. 2002; Anderson et al. 2002; Rowe and Shepherd 2002). All these studies report the use of a wide variety of involvement mechanisms and a general need by PCG/Ts to be seen to be doing something in this respect. However, most also point to difficulties in identifying specific outcomes that are clearly attributable to particular instances of involvement (a view particularly associated with non-PCT stakeholders in our study).

Thirdly, it is possible that strategies of public and patient involvement are only concerned with the needs and preferences of citizens and service users as a secondary issue. In an age where the lexicon of quality, accountability and transparency permeates swathes of public policy, might such a vocabulary be used by the government to enhance control over the medical profession – simultaneously the most powerful and autonomous professional element within the health service? The research reported here found that PCTs were beginning to oversee involvement at the level of individual general practices and, indeed, were including stipulations about user and public involvement in contractual agreements with their practices. Accordingly, public and patient involvement has to be seen from at least two perspectives in the future development of primary care within the NHS. First, public and patient involvement is just another issue among many about which primary care organizations have to demonstrate or feign active interest. Secondly, however, involvement may also constitute a point of reference in the tensions and strategies between four particular interests. These include a government concerned to modernize the NHS (partly through the mechanisms and ideology of surveillance and accountability), a new and increasingly assertive management at the level of PCTs, an autonomous and powerful (but increasingly defensive) medical profession, and a diverse collection of lay stakeholders who are no longer content to remain silent in debates on the future of the health service. Against this background it will, in future, be important to consider public and patient involvement not just in terms of the demonstrable impact of particular initiatives, but also as a rhetorical and strategic focus in debates and tensions around reform of the NHS.

Acknowledgements

The research on which this chapter is based was funded by the Department of Health as part of its 'Health in Partnership' initiative. Our thanks are due to

Dr Carolyn Davies and Dr Christine Farrell who managed the initiative, to all our respondents, to our co-investigators (Dr Philip Tovey and Professor Philip Heywood) and to the members of our project advisory group.

References

Alborz, A., Wilkin, D. and Smith, K. (2002) Are primary care groups and trusts consulting local communities?, *Health and Social Care in the Community*, 10(1): 20–7.

Allsop, J. and May, A. (1986) *The Emperor's New Clothes: Family Practitioner Committees in the 1980s*. London: King Edward's Hospital Fund for London.

Anderson, W. and Florin, D. (2000) *Involving the Public: One of Many Priorities*. London: King's Fund.

Anderson, W., Florin, D., Gillam, S. and Mountford, L. (2002) *Every Voice Counts: Primary Care Organisations and Public Involvement*. London: King's Fund.

Bond, M., Irving, L. and Cooper, C. (2001) *Public Involvement in Decision Making in Primary Care Groups*. Sheffield: University of Sheffield School of Health and Related Research.

Brown, I. (2000) Involving the public in general practice in an urban district: levels and type of activity and perceptions of obstacles, *Health and Social Care in the Community*, 8(4): 251–9.

Department of Health (1998a) *The New NHS: Modern and Dependable – Developing Primary Care Groups* (HSC 1998/139 and LAC(98)21). London: Department of Health.

Department of Health (1998b) *A First Class Service: Quality in the New NHS*. London: Department of Health.

Department of Health (1999) *Patient and Public Involvement in the New NHS*. London: Department of Health.

Department of Health (2001a) *Involving Patients and the Public in Health Care*. London: Department of Health.

Department of Health (2001b) *Patient Representation in the New NHS*. London: Department of Health.

Department of Health and Social Security (1970) *The Future Structure of the National Health Service* (The Crossman Green Paper). London: HMSO.

Dixon, J., Goodwin, N. and Mays, N. (1998) *Accountability of Total Purchasing Pilot Projects*. London: King's Fund.

Foot, M. (1973) *Aneurin Bevan 1945–1960*. London: Paladin.

Levitt, R. and Wall, A. (1984) *The Reorganized National Health Service*, 3rd edn. London: Croom Helm.

Milewa, T., Valentine, J. and Calnan, M. (1998) Managerialism and active citizenship in Britain's reformed health service: power and community in an era of decentralization, *Social Science and Medicine*, 47(4): 507–17.

Milewa, T., Dowswell, G. and Harrison, S. (2002a) Partnerships, power and the 'new' politics of community participation in British health care, *Social Policy and Administration*, 36(7): 796–809.

Milewa, T., Harrison, S., Ahmad, W. and Tovey, P. (2002b) Citizens' participation in primary health care planning: innovative citizenship practice in empirical perspective, *Critical Public Health*, 12(1): 39–53.

North, N. and Peckham, S. (2001) Analysing structural interests in primary care, *Social Policy and Administration*, 35(4): 426–40.

Rowe, R. and Shepherd, M. (2002) Public participation in the new NHS: no closer to citizen control?, *Social Policy and Administration*, 36(3): 275–90.

Royal Commission on Local Government (1969) *Royal Commission on Local Government: Report*. London: HMSO.

Royal Commission on the National Health Service (1979) *Royal Commission on the National Health Service: Report*. London: HMSO.

Secretary of State for Health (2000) *The NHS Plan: A Plan for Investment, A Plan for Reform*. London: The Stationery Office.

Transition Advisory Board for Patient and Public Involvement in Health (2002) *Progress Report, June 2002*. London: Department of Health.

Webster, C. (1988) *The Health Services Since the War: Vol. I. Problems of Health Care – the National Health Service before 1957*. London: HMSO.

12 Looking outwards

Primary care organizations and local partnerships

Caroline Glendinning, Anna Coleman and Kirstein Rummery

Introduction: partnerships – definitions and rationales

Since their creation in 1999, primary care groups and trusts (PCG/Ts) have been subject to repeated encouragement and exhortations to work in 'partnership' with other organizations and services. As Newman (2001) points out, 'attempts to create more joined-up government are not a new feature of public policy; there is a long-standing tradition of initiatives designed to bring about better integration of policies and services' (p. 105). However, partnerships have become a distinctive feature of current policies, both within the NHS and between the NHS and other organizations and sectors (Glendinning *et al.* 2002a).

At least three rationales for partnerships can be identified. Theoretically, they are strongly associated with assertions of the increasing fragmentation and complexity of public life and the corresponding need to govern through coordination and steering mechanisms, rather than more direct and hierarchical forms of control (Newman 2001; Clark 2002). Secondly, partnerships may offer 'added value' – opportunities to tackle complex social problems or achieve policy goals that cannot be met by individual services, agencies or sectors acting alone (Hastings 1996; Audit Commission 1998). For example, the establishment of Health Action Zones (Bauld and Judge 2002) and the 1998 Green Paper on health inequalities both explicitly acknowledged the multiple causes of poor health and the consequent need for coordinated cross-sectoral and inter-agency action: 'the strength and effectiveness of partnerships in driving local action will be the key to determining success' (Secretary of State for Health 1998: 39). Thirdly, partnerships may increase both the efficiency of services and the quality of users' experiences. This latter rationale underpins the increasingly narrow focus since 1997 on relationships between health and social care services in political discourse, policies and associated performance management regimes (Secretary of State for Health 2000, 2002). Health ministers have repeatedly called for improved collaboration to break down the alleged 'Berlin Wall' between health and social care, with threats of compulsion, financial penalties and, ultimately, enforced restructuring as the consequences of partnership 'failure' (Hudson and Henwood 2002). However, while there is an extensive body of literature on the processes of 'doing' partnerships (see, for example, Audit Commission 1998; Balloch and Taylor 2001; Glendinning *et al.* 2002a), there is still little evidence about whether the expected benefits of partnerships are realized or whether they might be outweighed by any costs.

'Partnership' is a term characterized by 'methodological anarchy and definitional chaos' (Ling 2000: 82). Inter-agency partnerships may need variously to tackle structural, procedural, financial, cultural and professional barriers (Hardy *et al.* 1992; Newman 2001; Clark 2002; Hudson 2002). For the purposes of this chapter, partnerships are located around the middle of a continuum of collaboration, which extends from 'separation' through 'encounter', 'communication' and 'collaboration' to full 'integration' (Hudson *et al.* 1997; 1999; Leutz 1999). Thus partner organizations exist as autonomous units with separate, internal structures and external accountabilities, but enter into areas of joint decision-making and take into account each other's actions and the consequences for the other partner when making their own decisions. Partnerships may have different implications for different elements of large, complex organizations; some may require the active engagement of middle managers or frontline staff; others may depend mainly on formal agreements between senior officers and/or governing boards.

In this chapter, we first describe briefly the history of relationships between primary care and other services. We then examine the development of partnerships between PCG/Ts and their respective local authorities, at strategic and operational levels. This examination includes the role of social services representatives on PCG/T boards and their potential and actual role in promoting inter-agency partnerships; the progress made by PCG/Ts and social services departments in commissioning and providing services together; and the development of relationships between PCG/Ts and a wider range of local authority services. In the final section, we consider some of the continuing barriers to partnerships experienced by PCG/Ts.

The chapter draws on two data sources. Quantitative data from the longitudinal Tracker Survey of PCG/Ts (Glendinning and Coleman 1999; Coleman and Glendinning 2001, 2002) is complemented with qualitative material from a linked, in-depth study, also carried out between 1999 and 2002, of partnerships between a subsample of four PCG/Ts and their respective local authorities. In the latter study, semi-structured interviews were carried out with a wide range of PCG/T and local authority managers and frontline practitioners

(Rummery and Coleman 2003; Coleman and Rummery, 2003). These latter interviews provided an opportunity to explore subjective perceptions and qualitative accounts of the development of partnerships between the two sectors.

The history of partnerships in primary care

The history of collaboration between health and other statutory services (especially social care) is at best mixed, but collaboration involving primary care has been particularly problematic. Until 1999, primary care services, especially those provided by general practitioners (GPs), were not integral elements of the larger National Health Service (NHS) organizational units – area health authorities (subsequently district health authorities) and NHS trusts – that were the natural partners for local authorities seeking to collaborate on area-wide assessments of need and provision of services. General practitioners and other practice-based professionals had little experience of collaboration, particularly over locality-level, strategic activities such as assessing needs, reviewing service provision and equitably directing new investment. General practitioners, whose perspectives dominated the early years of PCG/Ts, have traditionally been preoccupied with securing service improvements for the patients of their practices, regardless of wider policy or equity issues (see Chapter 5).

Moreover, the quasi-markets in health and social care during the 1990s emphasized competition and the exercise of purchasing leverage rather than collaboration, and increased fragmentation so that local authorities had to deal with a potentially large number of primary care purchasers and service commissioners. These developments increased the difficulties of managing complex, local inter-organizational networks (Wistow and Hardy 1996). Quasi-markets also prompted major internal restructuring, within both the NHS and local government, that disrupted the continuity and trust on which good collaborative relationships depend (Hiscock and Pearson 1999).

Before the establishment of PCG/Ts, most examples of collaboration between primary care and social services involved operational-level initiatives to improve communication between frontline staff, such as outposting social services care managers in GP surgeries or appointing 'link' workers to speed up referral and assessment processes (see Glendinning *et al.* 1998). General practitioner fundholders tended to use their purchasing power to buy social work services to relieve pressures on their own practice-based services (Rummery and Glendinning 2000). Even those total purchasing projects interested in developing community and continuing care services showed scant awareness of the wider community care policy agenda and little interest in collaborating with social services partners (Wyke *et al.* 1999).

Primary care groups/trusts and the new partnership agenda

The 1997 White Paper announced that all NHS organizations would be placed under a statutory duty to work in partnership, both with each other and with other organizations. To encourage this, each primary care group (PCG) and primary care trusts (PCI) was required to 'have a governing body which includes . . . social services' (Secretary of State for Health 1997: 36). In establishing their boundaries around 'natural communities', PCG/Ts were urged to 'take account also of the benefits of coterminosity with social services' (Secretary of State for Health 1997: 37). Health improvement plans provided a local framework for joint action on the wider social and environmental determinants of (ill)health. Although health authorities were to take the lead in preparing a health improvement plan, local authorities were expected to be active participants in developing and implementing the objectives of such plans.

Other contemporary announcements made it clear that collaboration 'was not simply back on the agenda, but was at the very heart of new policies on health and social care in the shape of "partnership"' (Hudson and Henwood 2002: 157). National Service Priorities were set for health and social services; these explicitly identified areas for joint working, particularly in relation to services for older and disabled people (Department of Health 1998a). New joint investment plans required joint commissioning of services for older people and people with disabilities or mental illness (Department of Health 2000b). Resources were earmarked in the Social Services Modernization Fund to foster partnerships between health and social services (Department of Health 1999a). A consultation document, *Partnership in Action* (Department of Health 1998b), followed by clauses in the 1999 Health Act, removed some of the structural obstacles that were perceived to impede joint working between NHS and local authority services.

This initially facilitative policy was quickly superseded by a much more directive approach, accompanied by further promises of carrots and threats of sticks. *The NHS Plan* (Secretary of State for Health 2000) announced the creation of new, completely integrated organizations – health and social care trusts – a 'new level' of PCT that commissions and/or provides social as well as health services, and indicated that care trusts would be imposed by the Secretary of State where 'local health and social organizations have failed to establish effective joint partnerships' (Secretary of State for Health 2000: 73). Two years later, additional funding for both NHS and local authority social services was made conditional on improved performance – including improvements in collaboration between NHS and social services organizations, as demonstrated by reduced numbers of delayed hospital discharges. Failures would be subject to financial penalties and further (unspecified) incentives were promised to encourage and reward joint activities (Secretary of State for Health 2002).

Given these pressures, an important indicator of PCG/Ts' 'success' in building partnerships is likely to be reflected in the joint commissioning and joint provision of services for older people and other groups with long-term, multiple service needs. However, the wider obligations of PCG/Ts to improve the health of local people, and those of local authorities to promote the well-being of their residents, have not diminished. Both obligations were originally located within the overarching framework of the health improvement plan – an 'important driving force in the enactment of the new duties imposed on the NHS and local government bodies' (Knight *et al.* 2001: 139). Subsequently, local strategic partnerships have offered a new, overarching framework for local partnerships. These are cross-agency, umbrella partnerships, led but not 'owned' by local authorities, which have a broad remit to improve the quality of life of local communities (Department of Environment, Transport and the Regions 2001). The involvement of PCG/Ts in these wider inter-sectoral partnerships, whose outcomes are likely to be long-term, diffuse and locality-specific, is discussed in Chapter 10.

The range of policies required to be delivered through local partnerships involving PCG/Ts suggests some potential tensions between the creation and strengthening of devolved, local organizational and service networks, and more directive, hierarchical forms of 'steering'. This is described by Newman (2001: 111) as the tension between the 'long-term agenda of addressing intractable problems with the need to retain control' over delivering the government's agenda. As this chapter will show, this tension characterizes the experiences of PCG/Ts in developing local partnerships.

The role of the social services representative

Given the poor history of health/social services collaboration, the inclusion on PCG/T boards of a representative from the local social services department offered new opportunities for 'encounters' that could potentially lead to 'communication' and perhaps eventually 'collaboration' (Hudson *et al.* 1997, 1999). Depending on the organizational and communication arrangements within their employing authorities, social services representatives could also facilitate linkages between the PCG/T and the functions and services of the wider local authority that impact upon the health and well-being of local communities. Early policy guidance recommended that these representatives should be managers with operational responsibilities (NHS Executive 1998a), perhaps reflecting an implicit assumption that the closer alignment of front-line services was the major partnership priority, or to maintain parity with GP and nursing members of the PCG/T board. However, many social services

Table 12.1 Responsibilities of social services representatives

Responsibilities	1999/2000		2000/1		2001/2	
	n	%	n	%	n	%
Mainly operational	5	10	6	14	4	7
Mainly strategic	16	31	14	33	21	39
Operational and strategic	29	57	19	44	26	48
Other	1	2	4	9	3	6

departments apparently ignored this advice and the majority of representatives (around 80 per cent) have consistently had at least some senior strategic management responsibilities (Table 12.1).

Initially, social services representatives found it difficult to feel involved in the activities of the board for several reasons. First, they suffered a substantial 'knowledge gap' about primary care, GPs and the role of the new PCG/Ts:

> I was starting from a very low knowledge base of GPs and how they worked and what drove them. It took me a while to actually understand them and understand what drove them in terms of how they function.
>
> (Social services representative, PCG board, case study site, year 1)

Conversely, other PCG board members admitted that they did not understand fully the functions and responsibilities of social services departments. However, this mutual lack of knowledge quickly showed marked improvement. The proportions of social services representatives reporting friendly and constructive attitudes on the part of other board members rose from 58 per cent in 1999 to 77 per cent the following year, as a result of the new opportunities for regular contact over PCG/T activities:

> I think there's been an enhancement of understanding and mutual respect, and I do think that's quite genuine. One of the biggest complaints you get from GPs is you can never get to see a social worker, never get hold of anyone and people are quite elusive, and I think the face-to-face contact breaks that barrier down, and they see these people and they can see that they're very professional and able, and I think that makes a big difference.
>
> (Health authority manager, case study site, year 2)

However, increased understanding and respect does not seem to have been accompanied by greater influence on the part of social services representatives within the activities of PCG/T boards and executive committees. Social services representatives holding positions of office on PCG/T boards have remained a very small minority. Social services representatives have also continued to report exercising less influence in PCG/T decision-making than other groups and interests represented on the board, a position that was confirmed by other stakeholders. In 1999, 54 per cent of PCG chief executives rated their social services representatives as having little or no influence, compared with only 5 per cent who rated GPs as having little or no influence. One year later, 44 per cent of PCG/T chief executives still rated social services representatives as having little or no influence. This may have reflected an early preoccupation of the board with internal organizational and clinical matters, to which social services representatives could make little contribution:

> I think there is a real issue with how the PCGs are manned [*sic*], with the chief officer and very little else. Quite recently [this locality] has received additional management support, but really their staffing has been inadequate in terms of the task, which has meant that they've therefore concentrated on health systems-type things and not on integration. But then, at their stage of development . . . [the priority was] meeting those problems before thinking about how to work with social services. And I think they were quite right.
> (Social services commissioning manager, case study site, year 1)

Other interviewees cited differences in professional values and orientations. Both social services and other non-NHS members of PCG/T boards pointed to GPs' traditional focus on patients and practice-level matters and the inappropriateness of this tradition for the kind of decision-making for which PCG/Ts were now responsible:

> What the GPs on the board are concerned about is what happens to their individual patients. I don't think they're quite evolved to the stage where they're thinking strategically yet, they're still focused, quite rightly in a lot of respects, on what this is going to mean for GPs in their practice and for their patients.
> (Social services representative, PCG Board, case study site, year 1)

Organizational turbulence also affects partnerships, as this disrupts continuity and the development of trust between key individuals (Hudson and Hardy 2002). There was a surprisingly high turnover among social services representatives serving on PCG/T boards. By early 2002, only 30 per cent of social services representatives had held that role since the establishment of the PCG in April 1999 and a further 32 per cent had only been appointed during the past year:

... our vice chair actually left and has gone to work in a different area and it took social services some time to, to actually get somebody else on the board ... There has been that inevitable gap.

(Chief executive, PCG, case study site, year 2)

Some of the turnover among social services representatives may reflect the changes within PCG/Ts as the latter have merged and/or become trusts. However, in 2002, 39 per cent of PCG/Ts with no history of mergers nevertheless still had social services representatives who had only come into post within the past year. This additional turnover may therefore also reflect the seniority of the social services representatives and the difficulties they reported in combining their work on the PCG/T board with their other departmental responsibilities.

Cementing partnerships: planning and providing services together

An important factor contributing to successful partnerships is the mutual recognition of the need to work together (as well as acknowledgement of those areas where collaboration is not necessary or appropriate) (Hudson and Hardy 2002). Indeed, the experience of working together can itself further deepen partners' appreciation of their interdependence. From 1999 onwards, a growing range of joint activities between PCG/Ts and social services developed, from strategic planning and commissioning down to the alignment of front-line services.

Partnerships in planning and commissioning

For the first year or so after the formation of PCGs, health authorities continued to take the NHS lead for most joint commissioning of services with social services. Even by 2000, only 11 per cent of PCG/Ts had taken over full responsibility for joint commissioning of older people's services with their social services counterparts and only 3 per cent of PCG/Ts were fully responsible for the joint commissioning of adult mental health or learning disability services. However, with the abolition of health authorities in 2002, joint commissioning responsibilities were rapidly transferred (Wilkin *et al.* 2002). By early 2002, between a half and three-quarters of PCG/Ts were involved in the joint commissioning of older people's services, learning disability services or adult mental health services. The range of older people's services that PCG/Ts were jointly commissioning with social services partners reflected national government priorities for intermediate care services, the most common being community-based rehabilitation schemes, joint care management, rapid response home care services and joint equipment services. The proportion of PCG/Ts involved in the investment of 'badged' Social Services Modernization Fund grants for carers' services, partnership, prevention and promoting independence (Department of Health 1999a) also increased steadily; by 2001/ 2, 96 per cent reported that social services partners were involving them in using these funds.

However, other evidence suggests that collaboration, particularly with social services, may still be marginal to some key areas of PCG/T activity, where traditional stakeholder interests remain highly influential. Arguably, commissioning integrated services requires contributions from a range of agencies and perspectives to ensure that patient pathways between services are clear and continuous (Audit Commission 2002). The breadth of consultation and stakeholder involvement could therefore constitute an indicator of a 'whole systems' approach to commissioning. Nevertheless, by 2000/1, a third of PCG/Ts still had no subgroup with specific responsibilities for commissioning hospital and community health services. In those that had, membership was heavily biased towards GPs (members of 94 per cent of commissioning subgroups) and community nurses (members of 58 per cent of commissioning groups). Other GP practice-based staff, community health service managers and clinicians, acute sector staff, other health professionals and lay people were far less well represented and only two-fifths of commissioning subgroups included a social services representative. This picture had changed little by the third Tracker Survey, which showed that GPs were represented on virtually all (95 per cent) commissioning subgroups, but still only 45 per cent had social services representation (Glendinning *et al.* 2001a; Coleman and Glendinning 2002).

Even if the membership of PCG/T commissioning groups represents only a narrow range of interests, this may be overcome if commissioning strategies are informed by consultation with relevant stakeholders. However, the second round of the Tracker Survey revealed that consultation to inform the commissioning of services was largely restricted to primary and community health professionals, and hospital clinicians and nurses in the case of acute services (Glendinning *et al.* 2001a). Social services were more likely to be consulted about the commissioning of community than acute health services, but even here nearly half of PCG/Ts reported no social services consultation. Not surprisingly, therefore, only one-fifth of PCG/T board members with lead responsibility for commissioning in 2002 considered that social services had any influence over commissioning decisions, while the influence of users, carers and their representative organizations was minimal. The lack of social services involvement in commissioning is perhaps surprising, given the high policy salience attached to the interface between hospitals and social services in preventing admissions and securing prompt discharge.

Joint activities

The creation of joint posts between PCG/Ts and local authorities is a further indicator of partnerships. By 2002, 58 per cent of PCG/Ts had a coordinator of intermediate care services jointly employed with the local authority and 70 per cent of PCG/Ts had other staff employed specifically to develop links between the PCG/T and its respective local authority:

> I think there's been a significant strengthening [in relations with social services] . . . Social services have actually appointed somebody to coordinate the work with PCTs across the . . . district. So he's been very helpful and then, we've continued with our work with the social services member, who is now on the professional executive committee, rather than the board.
>
> (Chief executive, PCT, case study site, year 2)

The 'flexibilities' contained in section 31 of the Health Act 1999 went 'live' in April 2000. The flexibilities remove some of the structural barriers to closer inter-agency collaboration and facilitate movement along the collaborative continuum towards full integration. They allow NHS organizations and local authorities to pool budgets for specific services, delegate commissioning responsibilities to a single 'lead' organization and employ health and social care staff within the same organization. As subcommittees of their health authorities, PCGs did not have the appropriate status to be statutory signatories to such partnerships, although many of the early partnerships using the flexibilities did nevertheless involve their local PCG/Ts (Glendinning *et al.* 2002c). However, by early 2002, as more PCGs had become trusts and the remainder anticipated shortly doing so, over half reported they currently had one or more service partnerships using the Health Act flexibilities.

Frontline partnerships

If users are to experience 'seamless' services, better collaboration at operational and frontline levels is also required. This might involve relocating staff, so that health and social care staff are based in the same premises or in integrated teams; providing joint training; changing staff roles and responsibilities to reduce duplication and gaps in skills; seconding staff to another organization under a single, integrated management; and introducing common procedures (for example, in relation to assessment) across organizational and professional boundaries. By the third round of the Tracker Survey in 2002 (Coleman and Glendinning 2002), initiatives such as these involving front-line health and social care staff were widespread (Figure 12.1).

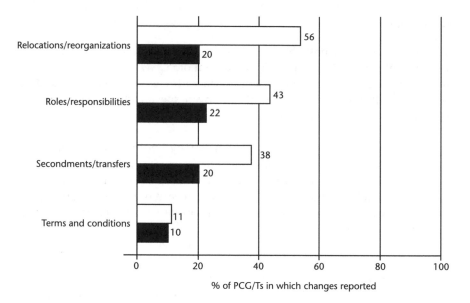

Figure 12.1 Changes in health/social services staff. ▢, 2001/2; ■, 2001/1.

By 2002, 42 per cent of PCG/Ts said that social workers were attached to their GP surgeries or that GP link/liaison workers were in post. Far fewer PCG/Ts reported changes in the terms and conditions of employment of health and social care staff than other staffing changes. Changes to terms and conditions of employment are likely to be more difficult than other personnel changes to negotiate and agree with staff and their representative organizations. It may be that many PCG/Ts are, therefore, attempting to maximize other opportunities for closer collaboration between frontline practitioners instead. Indeed, by 2002, most PCG/Ts (89 per cent) reported recent joint training activities between their own and local authority staff, including training about the new single assessment process.

Wider inter-agency partnerships

Official guidance on the role of social services representatives suggested that they may be able to act as a gateway to other local government departments such as environmental health, housing and education (NHS Executive 1998b). Early evidence suggested that social services representatives were indeed crucially important in developing robust communications and other relationships between the PCG/T and the wider social services department and local authority (Glendinning et al. 2001b). In both 1999 and 2000, around four-fifths of social services representatives reported meeting regularly with their

department's senior management team or senior officer group to discuss PCG/
T matters; 21 per cent met regularly with local councillors and 15 per cent with
divisional or team leaders about PCG/T developments. A substantial minority
of social services representatives also communicated regularly with frontline
colleagues by, for example, holding regular meetings with divisional officers or
circulating PCG/T board minutes to the social services teams within the PCG/T
boundary.

However, social services representatives have not been the only means by
which PCG/Ts have 'encountered' and 'communicated with' a wider range of
local authority services. From their earliest days, PCG/Ts adopted several strategies for developing such links (Glendinning *et al.* 2001b). In 1999, the social
services representatives on a fifth of all PCG/T boards came from authorities in
which their department was combined with another local authority service
function such as housing, leisure and recreation or community development.
In theory, this could facilitate representation of these wider interests. Social
services representatives themselves often had wider, health-related responsibilities, such as contributing to the Joint Investment Plan or representing their
department in health improvement plan discussions. A third strategy was for
PCG/Ts to co-opt other local authority representatives onto their boards and
by 2000 a third had done so. These additional co-optees were twice as likely to
be local authority officers as elected councillors.

The PCG/Ts also quickly developed collaborative relationships with a wide
range of other local authority departments. By 2000, only 12 per cent of PCG/
Ts reported no such wider local authority collaborations. By 2002, all PCG/Ts
were collaborating with their respective local authorities on community
development/urban regeneration issues and most had established other inter-
sectoral collaborations as well. These, and PCG/T involvement in wider, multi-
agency, locality-based initiatives, are reported in more detail in Chapter 10.
However, it is important to note that, as well as indicating PCG/T engagement
in local partnerships, these fora also provided opportunities for regular
contacts between senior officers and managers, thereby helping to cement
relationships between the leaders on whom successful partnerships depend
(Hudson and Hardy 2002).

In addition, by 2002, 45 per cent of PCG/Ts reported having developed at
least one partnership with a private sector provider. These partnerships most
frequently involved capital development schemes, pharmaceutical companies
providing staff training, and intermediate- and long-term care services based
in private sector nursing and care homes.

The integrated funding streams for which PCG/Ts are responsible offer
opportunities for shifting resources and expenditure priorities from traditional
areas of investment. By 2002, 85 per cent of PCG/Ts were allocating resources
to non-NHS initiatives aimed at improving health or quality of life and two-
thirds were contributing to at least three such initiatives; these were most

likely to be community development projects (76 per cent), services to support family carers (72 per cent) and accident prevention initiatives (64 per cent).

In the future, relationships between local authorities and PCG/Ts will be underpinned by the new powers of local authorities to scrutinize the work of local NHS services and organizations (Department of Health 2002). These powers both allow PCG/Ts to be held to account by local elected councillors and enable the plans of local NHS organizations to be integrated into the overarching strategic umbrella of local strategic partnerships. Although the new scrutiny powers did not come into force until January 2003, almost all the PCTs that took part in the 2002 Tracker Survey had already held discussions with their respective local authorities about this new function (Coleman and Glendinning 2002; see also Chapter 11). Most were positive about the potential for complementing the other partnership activities of the PCT board, as were interviewees in the four case study sites:

> . . . we've picked out some key elements for discussion – around rules of engagement, styles of working, particularly reviews, development needs and also trying to look at the resource implication from both sides – hopefully out of that a multidisciplinary project group will work through the summer leading up to an agreed programme of reviews and we're going to have sort of like a test run in the autumn.
> (Social services representative on PCT board, site C, year 3)

Partnership problems and barriers

The development of these external relationships by PCG/Ts has taken place against a background of very considerable organizational turbulence as, over only 3 years, PCGs have become full-fledged trusts and many have merged with their neighbours (see Chapter 6). Such changes can divert organizational attention from the development of external relationships and disrupt the interpersonal relationships between key individuals on whom external partnerships depend. It is therefore not surprising that a third of the social services representatives responding to the Tracker Survey in both 2001 and 2002 cited organizational turbulence and change as major barriers to partnerships (Coleman and Glendinning 2001, 2002).

Local authorities also underwent restructuring over the same period. The Local Government Act 2000 required them to amend their decision-making structures and most have reorganized their departmental-based committees to a simple executive (decision-making) and scrutiny (overseeing) distinction. Some have undertaken other internal restructuring, particularly of their social services functions, to improve the alignment of their day-to-day service operations with the boundaries of local PCG/Ts. For example, one of the case study sites planned to restructure its social work services to make its older people's teams coterminous with the PCT boundaries.

Nevertheless, different cartographical boundaries between PCG/Ts and local authorities have remained a major barrier to partnerships. From their earliest days, a third of PCG/Ts had responsibility for patients who lived outside the boundaries of the social services department from which the social services representative on the board was drawn (Glendinning and Coleman 1999). Subsequent mergers between PCG/Ts did not appear to address these boundary differences. According to the 2000/1 Tracker Survey, in only a fifth of PCG/Ts did the desire to align boundaries or achieve better coordination with local authority services feature as a reason for planned mergers and/or becoming a trust (Coleman and Glendinning 2001). By 2002, boundary differences were still cited as an obstacle to closer partnerships by a fifth of PCG/Ts (Coleman and Glendinning 2002).

Finally, both PCG/Ts and local authorities remain subject to an extensive range of national priorities that divert attention from, and may even occasionally undermine, external collaborative relationships:

> It has been difficult, keeping the health and health service agenda going particularly in the early days, because we were . . . running the risk of putting enormous demands on the clinicians in shaping services for the future when they were very busy. Primary care professionals are only just beginning to come to terms with the changes around clinical governance and in a structured way, being part of the PCT . . . .
>
> (Health authority manager, case study site, year 2)

These priorities, which form the basis of the separate performance management systems for PCG/Ts and local authorities respectively, have both restricted the capacity of PCG/Ts to develop partnerships and shaped the focus of the partnerships that have developed:

> . . . our local social services department has been very heavily squeezed recently because, you know education is top of the list, and children's services, in this local authority, in common with many others. So it did look for a while as if social services funding was going to become a major issue and that they weren't going to have enough money . . . We all recognize at the end of the day we have to meet our waiting list targets.
>
> (Chief executive, PCT board, case study site, year 2)

Moreover, many areas of partnership activity – especially the joint commissioning and provision of services – appeared to be determined primarily by national priorities such as the national service frameworks (Department of Health 1999b, 2000a, 2001) and *The NHS Plan* (Secretary of State for Health 2000). This suggests a potential tension between more hierarchical modes of policy implementation and the local ownership and commitment that are likely to sustain local collaboration (Rummery 2002).

Conclusions

In view of the poor history of collaboration between primary care and social services, the range of relationships and joint activities that have developed between the two sectors is an undoubted success. The early encounters between social services representatives and the other members of PCG/T boards, characterized by a degree of suspicion and hostility, reflected this history. These encounters also reflected long-standing differences in organizational forms between the sectors, with social services representatives apparently finding it easier to engage with the corporate and strategic agendas of the new primary care organizations than GPs, who were more familiar with safeguarding the interests of their smaller practice and patient populations.

However, from initially constituting the foundation on which to build wider inter-sectoral partnerships, the presence of social services representatives on PCG/T boards has rapidly been complemented by a wide range of local inter-organizational networks. The PCG/Ts now appear to be engaging in collaborative commissioning with social services counterparts, especially in high-profile policy areas like intermediate care and other services for older people. Conversely, social services are involving PCG/Ts in new investments using 'badged' Social Services Modernization funds. The PCG/Ts have also developed mechanisms for liaising with a range of other local authority departments and services, independent of the channel offered by the social services representative. The engagement of PCG/Ts with wider, multi-agency networks and initiatives is also striking (see also Chapter 10). The fact that these partnerships have developed in a context of unprecedented organizational turbulence within both the NHS and local government is particularly remarkable. The development of PCGs' own internal organizational capacity in preparation for the rapid transition to trust status and the acquisition in 2002 of many former health authority responsibilities (see Chapter 6) constituted a major distraction from building and sustaining their external relationships. Moreover, these PCG/T–local authority partnerships have developed despite continuing differences in geographical boundaries. Opportunities to improve boundary alignments in the course of PCG/T mergers appear largely to have been overlooked and these therefore continue to be perceived locally as barriers to inter-sectoral partnerships.

New relationships between organizations need to be translated into new ways of working at operational and frontline levels, if service users are to experience more 'joined up', seamless services; new organizational structures do not automatically overcome the inter-professional differences between primary health and social care workers (Withington and Giller 2001; Hudson 2002). Here again PCG/Ts and their social services partners appear to have made progress, at least in addressing the 'soft' human resource issues – attitudes, culture and day-to-day working practices – associated with building partnerships. Joint training, co-location and integrated health and social care staff teams may all, in time, help to break down the professional 'tribalisms' that can impede top-down partnership initiatives. The impact of changes to professional organization and practice on the ways that services are delivered to users is likely to take some time to become apparent.

However, some aspects of the structure and functions of the new PCTs may, in the long run, inhibit collaboration and partnerships. First, the governance arrangements of PCTs reflect several different, sometimes competing, stakeholder interests. Some of these interests, particularly those of GPs and other clinicians, may continue to exert disproportionate influence over PCT activities. The widespread absence of involvement or consultation with social services partners in the commissioning of hospital and, to a lesser extent, community health services reflects these inequalities, as does the continuing relative lack of influence of social services representatives in PCT decision-making.

Moreover, the focus of PCT activities, including those involving collaboration with local authority partners, continues to be dominated by national policy priorities. In many areas, health and social care services have a long history of collaboration in relation to learning disability or mental health services (Glendinning *et al.* 2002c; Peck *et al.* 2002a, b) and this might be expected to offer a solid foundation on which further organizational learning can be built. However, it is older people's services, as mandated by *The NHS Plan* and related policy imperatives, that provide the focus of much current collaboration. Moreover, the older people's services that are the current focus of partnerships are those prioritized and targeted with 'badged' funding by central government – short-term intermediate care and other intensive interventions to avoid delayed hospital discharge, rather than a wider range of longer-term, preventive services as urged by the older people's national service framework (Department of Health 2001; Glendinning *et al.* 2002b).

The dominance of high-profile national policy issues within PCG/T partnerships has several consequences that may prove unhelpful for the longer-term sustainability of those partnerships. First, it may be difficult for PCG/Ts and local authorities to create and maintain strong local ownership and involvement in collaborative activities and build trust at all levels between their organizations, if these essential attributes of successful partnerships

(Hudson and Hardy 2002) are eclipsed by pressures to respond to national policy imperatives and meet nationally imposed service targets. It may also be difficult to sustain the notion of partnerships as characteristic of devolved, networked modes of governance, rather than traditional top-down bureaucratic modes of delivering welfare (Rhodes 1997).

This risk is increased if the national policy targets that local partnerships are to address reflect issues that have traditionally been the concern of one, rather than both, partner organizations. Such inequalities of interest are not automatically incompatible within local partnerships, so long as all partners concur with the unequal distribution of inputs, costs or benefits. However, the terms of the national policy debate – especially the creation of completely integrated health and social care trusts – have led to suspicions that the interests and expertise of social services are increasingly subordinated to those of the NHS (Hudson and Henwood 2002). Such parameters are not conducive to the establishment of trust between local partners.

Moreover, national policy priorities risk marginalizing the very partnerships in which PCG/Ts are making the most unexpected progress – those with other local authority services, community organizations and multi-agency initiatives (see Chapter 10). Again, the history of primary health services (especially general practice) contributions to such enterprises is not promising. However, the extensive range of such collaborations developed by PCG/Ts within their first few years, combined with the financial contributions that many are making to non-NHS services, reflect a commitment to improving the quality of life and reducing health inequalities among local people. Of course, the benefits of such initiatives are likely to be long-term, diffuse and difficult to capture in performance indicators or quality targets. It will be important for central government to give due recognition to these initiatives and ensure that they constitute part of any future assessment of the collaborative capacity of PCTs.

References

Audit Commission (1998) *A Fruitful Partnership*. London: The Audit Commission.
Audit Commission (2002) *Integrated Services for Older People: Building a Whole System Approach in England*. London: The Audit Commission.
Balloch, S. and Taylor, M. (eds) (2001) *Partnership Working: Policy and Practice?* Bristol: The Policy Press.
Bauld, L. and Judge, K. (eds) (2002) *Learning from Health Action Zones*. Chichester: Aeneas Press.
Clark, T. (2002) New Labour's big idea: joined up government, *Social Policy and Society*, 1(2): 107–17.
Coleman, A. and Glendinning, C. (2001) Partnerships, in D. Wilkin, S. Gillam

and A. Coleman (eds) *The National Tracker Survey of Primary Care Groups and Trusts 2000/2001: Modernising the NHS?* Manchester: The University of Manchester.

Coleman, A. and Glendinning, C. (2002) Partnerships, in D. Wilkin, A. Coleman, B. Dowling and K. Smith (eds) *The National Tracker Survey of Primary Care Groups and Trusts 2001/2002: Taking Responsibility?* Manchester: The University of Manchester.

Coleman, A. and Rummery, K. (2003) Social service representation in primary care groups and trusts, *Journal of Interprofessional Care*, 17(3): 273–80.

Department of Environment, Transport and the Regions (2001) *Local Strategic Partnerships: Government Guidance*. London: DETR.

Department of Health (1998a) *Modernising Health and Social Services: National Priorities Guidance*. London: Department of Health.

Department of Health (1998b) *Partnership in Action*. London: Department of Health.

Department of Health (1999a) *Modernising Social Services: Promoting Independence, Improving Protection, Raising Standards*. London: The Stationery Office.

Department of Health (1999b) *National Service Framework for Mental Health: Modern Standards and Service Models*. London: Department of Health.

Department of Health (2000a) *National Service Framework for Coronary Heart Disease: Modern Standards and Service Models*. London: Department of Health.

Department of Health (2000b) *Guidance on Joint Investment Plans* (downloaded from www.doh.gov.uk/jointunit, 12 January 2000).

Department of Health (2001) *National Service Framework for Older People: Modern Standards and Service Models*. London: Department of Health.

Department of Health (2002) *Delivering the NHS Plan: Next Steps on Investment, Next Steps on Reform*. London: Department of Health.

Glendinning, C. (2002) Partnerships between health and social services: developing a framework for evaluation, *Policy and Politics*, 30(1): 115–27.

Glendinning, C. and Coleman, A. (1999) Partnerships with local authorities, in D. Wilkin, S. Gillam and B. Leese (eds) *The National Tracker Survey of Primary Care Groups and Trusts: Progress and Challenges 1999/2000*. Manchester: The University of Manchester.

Glendinning, C., Rummery, K. and Clarke, R. (1998) From collaboration to commissioning: developing relationships between primary health and social services, *British Medical Journal*, 317 (7151): 122–5.

Glendinning, C., Coleman, A., Shipman, C. and Malbon, G. (2001a) Progress in partnerships, *British Medical Journal*, 323(7303): 28–31.

Glendinning, C., Abbott, S. and Coleman, A. (2001b) Bridging the gap: new relationships between primary care groups and local authorities, *Social Policy and Administration*, 35(4): 411–25.

Glendinning, C., Powell, M. and Rummery, K. (eds) (2002a) *Partnerships, New Labour and the Governance of Welfare*. Bristol: The Policy Press.

Glendinning, C., Coleman, A. and Rummery, K. (2002b) Partnerships, performance and primary care: developing integrated services for older people in England, *Ageing and Society*, 22(2): 185–208.

Glendinning, C., Hudson, B., Hardy, B. and Young, R. (2002c) *National Evaluation of Notifications for Use of the Section 31 Partnership Flexibilities in the Health Act 1999: Final Project Report*. Manchester: National Primary Care Research and Development Centre/Leeds: Nuffield Institute for Health.

Hardy, B., Turrell, A. and Wistow, G. (1992) *Innovations in Community Care Management*. Aldershot: Avebury.

Hastings, A. (1996) Unravelling the process of 'partnership' in urban regeneration policy, *Urban Studies*, 33(2): 253–68.

Hiscock, J. and Pearson, M. (1999) Looking inwards, looking outwards: dismantling the 'Berlin Wall' between health and social services?, *Social Policy and Administration*, 33(2): 150–63.

Hudson, B. (2002) Interprofessionality in health and social care: the Achilles' heel of partnership?, *Journal of Interprofessional Care*, 16(1): 7–17.

Hudson, B. and Hardy, B. (2002) What is a 'successful' partnership and how can it be measured?, in C. Glendinning, M. Powell and K. Rummery (eds) *Partnerships, New Labour and the Governance of Welfare*. Bristol: The Policy Press.

Hudson, B. and Henwood, M. (2002) The NHS and social care: the final countdown?, *Policy and Politics*, 30(2): 153–66.

Hudson, B., Hardy, B., Henwood, M. and Wistow, G. (1997) *Inter-agency Collaboration: Final Report*. Leeds: Nuffield Institute for Health, University of Leeds.

Hudson, B., Exworthy, M., Peckham, S. and Callaghan, G. (1999) *Locality Partnerships: The Early Primary Care Group Experience*. Leeds: Nuffield Institute for Health, University of Leeds.

Knight, T., Smith, J. and Cropper, S. (2001) Developing sustainable collaboration: learning from theory and practice, *Primary Health Care Research and Development*, 2: 139–48.

Leutz, W. (1999) Five laws for integrating medical and social services: lessons from the United States and the United Kingdom, *Millbank Quarterly*, 77(1): 77–110.

Ling, T. (2000) Unpacking partnership: the case of health care, in J. Clarke, S. Gewirtz and E. McLaughlin (eds) *New Managerialism, New Welfare?* London: Sage Publications.

Newman, J. (2001) *Modernising Governance: New Labour, Policy and Society*. London: Sage Publications.

NHS Executive (1998a) The *New NHS: Modern and Dependable. Establishing Primary Care Groups*, Health Service Circular 1998/065. Leeds: NHS Executive.

NHS Executive (1998b) The *New NHS: Modern and Dependable. Developing Primary Care Groups*, Local Authority Circular LAC(98)21. Leeds: NHS Executive.

Peck, E., Gulliver, P. and Towell, D. (2002a) Governance of partnership between health and social services: the experience in Somerset, *Health and Social Care in the Community*, 10(5): 331–8.

Peck, E., Gulliver, P. and Towell, D. (2002b) *Modernising Partnerships: An Evaluation of Somerset's Innovations in the Commissioning and Organisation of Mental Health Services*. London: King's College, Institute for Applied Health and Social Policy.

Rhodes, R. (1997) *Understanding Governance*. Buckingham: Open University Press.

Rummery, K. (2002) Towards a theory of welfare partnerships, in C. Glendinning, M. Powell and K. Rummery (eds) *Partnerships, New Labour and the Governance of Welfare*. Bristol: The Policy Press.

Rummery, K. and Coleman, A. (2003) Partners in care? Towards the development of joint and integrated primary health and social care services for older people, *Social Science and Medicine*.

Rummery, K. and Glendinning, C. (2000) *Primary Care and Social Services: Developing New Partnerships for Older People*. Oxford: Radcliffe Medical Press.

Secretary of State for Health (1997) *The New NHS: Modern, Dependable*, London: The Stationery Office.

Secretary of State for Health (1998) *Our Healthier Nation: A Contract for Health* London: The Stationery Office.

Secretary of State for Health (2000) *The NHS Plan: A Plan for Investment, A Plan for Reform*. London: The Stationery Office.

Secretary of State for Health (2002) *Delivering the NHS Plan: Next Steps on Investment, Next Steps on Reform*. London: The Stationery Office.

Wistow, G. and Hardy, B. (1996) Competition, collaboration and markets, *Journal of Interprofessional Care*, 10(1): 5–10.

Wilkin, D., Coleman, A., Dowling, B. and Smith, K. (eds) (2002) *The National Tracker Survey of Primary Care Groups and Trusts 2001/2002: Taking Responsibility?* Manchester: The University of Manchester.

Withington, S. and Giller, H. (2001) Multidisciplinary working and the new NHS: more messages from Northern Ireland, *Managing Community Care*, 8(6): 24–9.

Wyke, S., Myles, S., Popay, J., Scott, J., Campbell, A. and Girling, J. (1999) Total purchasing, community and continuing care: lessons for future policy developments in the NHS, *Health and Social Care in the Community*, 7(6): 394–407.

PART 3
Conclusions

PART 3
Conclusion

13 The 'new' primary care
Ideology and performance

Bernard Dowling and Caroline Glendinning

Introduction

The election of the Labour government in 1997 triggered a period of intense change within the National Health Service (NHS). Reflected in the title of the White Paper outlining the government's plans for the NHS, *The New NHS: Modern, Dependable* (Secretary of State for Health 1997), the term 'modernization' has increasingly been used to describe this transformation. However, this term is ambiguous and problematic. Its commonsense meaning assumes that agreement can be reached about what constitutes being 'up-to-date' or 'behind the times'. Simple definitions like this may be inappropriate when applied to a complex organizational, professional and political institution like the English NHS; in this context, the meaning of 'modernization' is likely to be both multidimensional and contested. In this book, 'modernization' is understood to signify the continuing search for improved performance and responsiveness, within clear budgetary limits. The process of 'modernization', as described in the preceding chapters, also appears to involve an intensification of regulatory mechanisms (including new mechanisms to regulate and restrict spending on and by primary care) and, significantly, the active involvement and incorporation of professional groups and networks within these enhanced regulatory regimes to a far greater extent than before (Newman 2001).

The main questions that arise from this 'modernization' programme concern the methods being used to change the NHS, the rationale behind these changes and the likelihood that they will be successful (or otherwise). These issues have constituted the central themes of this book.

The 'modernization' of the NHS locates primary care in a central position. Primary care has been charged both with transforming itself – the services provided by and within general practice and community health services – and with transforming the NHS as a whole. Indeed, the 'modernizing' task that has been set for primary care extends even beyond the traditional organizational boundaries of the NHS, which has to date been largely concerned with the treatment or management of ill-health, to a new responsibility for improving health and reducing inequalities in health. Fundamental to all these changes has been the establishment of primary care groups (PCGs) in 1999 and their progression since to primary care trusts (PCTs).

As happens with most incoming governments, these organizations, their responsibilities and, indeed, their intended impact on the NHS as a whole have all been branded 'new'. This claim corresponds with the rhetoric in the 1997 White Paper *The New NHS: Modern, Dependable* (Secretary of State for Health 1997) that Labour's policies for the NHS constitute a 'Third Way' that draws eclectically and pragmatically on, but does not slavishly follow, earlier models and structures. However, as Chapters 1, 2, 5 and 9 showed, many of the principles and practices reflected in the creation of primary care groups and trusts (PCG/Ts) draw heavily on the experiences of previous NHS models, particularly those of the internal market, general practitioner (GP) fundholding and total purchasing. Even within the government's own terms, it may be difficult to sustain the argument that the 'Third Way' NHS is fundamentally 'new'.

In this chapter, we first discuss what the 'Third Way' NHS means in the context of PCG/Ts. We then weigh up the evidence, presented in the contributions to this book, of how PCG/Ts have performed to date in meeting the expectations and demands that have been placed upon them. Finally, we speculate on the longer-term prospects for PCTs as the vehicle for NHS 'modernization'.

What counts and what is supposed to work

As Chapter 1 pointed out, assessing the performance and potential success of PCG/Ts is not easy, given the extensive and multidimensional nature of their responsibilities, the numerous targets and longer-term goals they have been set, and the many external factors likely to intervene and impact on their outcomes. Moreover, evaluating success can involve both intrinsic and extrinsic criteria; indeed, some criteria may fall into both categories. For example, improving health is one of the government's own (intrinsic) objectives for PCG/Ts, but the efficient contribution of any healthcare system to improving health is also likely to be an important element of any external (extrinsic) evaluation as well. Further distinctions could be made between the (summative) assessment of whether end-point outcomes (such as improving health) have been achieved and (formative) interim targets that reflect specific strategies or measures that are likely to achieve those objectives.

In this section, we consider whether PCG/Ts are likely to 'work' by examining them as examples of the government's proclaimed 'Third Way' in managing the state and its welfare services. The 'Third Way' in the NHS has pragmatic foundations. Both the 'Third Way' and the phrase 'what counts is what works' appear as subtitles in the same section – indeed, on the same page – of the 1997 White Paper (Secretary of State for Health 1997: 10). The implicit rejection of ideologically rooted approaches to health policy contains echoes of the 'end of ideology' ideas associated with much earlier political thinkers, such as Crosland (1956); it also raises the question of how far this avowed pragmatism itself has significant implicit ideological dimensions.

The government's 'Third Way' pragmatism in relation to its policies for the NHS allows it to draw eclectically on previous policies and models, as well as adding some new ones of its own. Political scientists have delineated three main 'ideal type' modes of governance: hierarchies, markets and networks (Thompson *et al.* 1991). Each denotes (among other things) differences in the nature of the relationships between the central state and its institutions and agents. Hierarchies are usually illustrated by the traditional top-down bureaucratic approach to the management of the NHS, with relationships between super- and subordinate levels legitimated by authority. Markets employ competition, contracts and a range of other financial mechanisms to achieve desired outcomes. Networks involve collaboration between broadly equal partners, in which self-regulation and trust play important roles.

Despite rejecting both the 'old centralised command and control systems of the 1970s' and the 'divisive internal market system of the 1990s' (Secretary of State for Health 1997: 10), the evidence presented in this book shows that Labour's policies for the NHS in fact contain very substantial elements of both, as well as significant aspects of the third mode of governance, that of networks. As Bond and Le Grand proposed in Chapter 2, the 'Third Way' sits between, or transcends, the twin dichotomies of private and public ownership and of hierarchical and market governance structures. Despite the development of private finance initiatives in the NHS, the governance dichotomy has been more apparent than that of the ownership of resources. The rejection of either a pure hierarchy or a pure market was clearly stated in *The NHS Plan*: 'Until the 1990s the NHS was run hierarchically with little room for local innovation or independence. In the 1990s the internal market introduced competition but failed to bring improvements. A new model is needed' (Secretary of State for Health 2000: 30).

However, far from rejecting these dominant modes of governance, the 'new' model involves combining very significant elements of both. A single page of *The NHS Plan* (Secretary of State for Health 2000: 30) asserts that 'standards cannot simply be set locally . . . Inspection, incentives, information and intervention, operating under the umbrella of clear national standards, will help reshape services around the patient'. However, the very same page also asserts that the 'NHS cannot be run from Whitehall' and that greater authority and decision-making powers need to be devolved to frontline staff: 'clinicians and managers want the freedom to run local services. They want to be able to shape services around patients' needs'. These multiple – and not entirely consistent – themes were also firmly reiterated in *Shifting the Balance of Power in the NHS* (Department of Health 2001).

The evidence presented in this book confirms that the establishment, operation and performance of PCG/Ts contain very substantial elements of both hierarchies and markets. Many of the chapters in Part 2 of the book describe the intensification of performance management regimes, tighter budgetary frameworks, inspections and targets – all forms of 'upward' accountability to central government that characterize hierarchical forms of governance. Indeed, the accelerated progression of PCGs to PCTs may itself reflect an urgency to ensure that these new organizations, with their very substantial financial responsibilities, could be more closely monitored and managed through mainstream NHS accountability structures. However, contributors also describe the continuing separation between the purchasers and providers of hospital services, the continuing use of contracts (albeit with important dimensions of service quality now included), and increases in the use of financial targets and incentives – market-related modes of influencing behaviours – both by central government and by PCTs in an attempt to influence the behaviours of their constituent practices and clinicians. This latter, quasi-market mode of governance can be expected to gain ascendancy with the proposed new GP contract and its extensive use of quality-related incentive payments.

In addition, in contrast to the adversarial nature of the former internal market, PCG/Ts have been explicitly expected to develop collaborative, partnership relationships with other public sector agencies. The partnership imperative (albeit mandated by central government) is a distinctive feature of Labour's policies (Glendinning *et al.* 2002) and reflects a more horizontal, networked mode of governance. Partnerships, between both agents and agencies, involve joint decision-making, the combination of expertise and the sharing of resources (including the resources of knowledge and capacity), in the quest for synergy and 'seamless' services for the user.

The rhetoric of the 'modernized' NHS refers repeatedly to the strengthened decision-making powers of frontline NHS staff (meaning local professionals, including doctors and nurses). This continues, and extends, the principal–agent relationships of the internal market, in which GPs purchased, or advised on the purchasing of, services on behalf their patients (Chapter 5). This theme was firmly reiterated in *Shifting the Balance of Power in the NHS* (Department of Health 2001), with the announcement that all PCGs would become PCTs by 2002 and that health authorities were to be abolished. However, as the preceding chapters show, the powers and freedoms that have been devolved to 'frontline professionals' (or, at least, those that are represented on professional executive committees of PCTs) are tightly circumscribed and are subject to the same targets, standards and inspection systems as the organizations to which they now belong. As Rose (1996) points out, these processes help to construct new forms of professional self-regulation, rendering professional decisions 'visible, calculable and amenable to evaluation' (p. 351). The new powers of PCTs – especially their responsibilities for very substantial tranches of public expenditure – have therefore been accompanied by substantial new responsibilities and accountabilities on behalf of the professionals who work within, and govern, them. Chapters 2 and 5, in particular, point to some of the potential flaws that may undermine this apparent devolution of NHS governance to local levels.

The NHS Plan also promised greater public participation in the governance of the NHS: the 'patient's voice does not sufficiently influence the provision of services', so giving 'patients new powers in the NHS is one of the keys to unlocking patient-centred services' (Secretary of State for Health 2000: 30). However, as Milewa and colleagues point out in Chapter 11, the creation of new opportunities for dialogues of different kinds to take place between PCTs, publics and patients may actually serve to restrict these to a limited number of prescribed and, therefore, legitimate channels. Opportunities to enhance the 'downward', local accountability of PCTs may therefore also have been circumscribed.

The 'modernized' NHS can, therefore, be characterized as a service in which the features of all three models of governance are present, possible and sometimes required. Targets and performance standards are set by central government and imposed on local organizations (hierarchies); the commissioners and providers of services are organizationally distinct and financial incentives and penalties are used to promote or penalize desired outcomes (markets); and collaboration by professionals within PCTs and between PCTs and other local agencies is encouraged (networks).

Evaluating performance: the tasks of primary care groups/ trusts

Given this eclectic combination of different modes of governance, to what extent are PCTs likely to deliver the 'modernization' of the NHS? In this section, the core tasks and responsibilities of PCG/Ts are set against the theoretical analyses and empirical evidence presented in this book. The starting point is the three core functions of PCG/Ts: to improve the health of people and reduce health inequalities; to develop primary and community health services; and to commission secondary health services. However, these functions are unlikely to be achieved unless certain other conditions are met. First, there is the organizational strength and capacity of PCG/Ts; unless they are 'fit' to meet the demands on them they will fail, as will the 'modernization' of the NHS as a whole. Organizational capacity includes the development of systems to manage consistent, high-quality information, which is central to both the development of effective local services and the monitoring of their performance. Secondly, some of the core functions of PCG/Ts (particularly those relating to health improvement and the development of integrated primary and community health services) depend on effective partnership working by PCG/Ts. Thirdly, PCG/Ts need to be able to meet the requirements for accountability, both 'upwards' to health authorities and central government and 'downwards' to local patients and publics.

Improving health and reducing health inequalities

The new responsibilities of PCG/Ts for improving health and reducing health inequalities represent significant shifts in the focus of primary care and, indeed, the NHS as a whole. General practitioners – the cornerstone of primary care – have traditionally been concerned with the treatment of illnesses among the small populations registered with their practices. Primary care trusts are required to focus on much larger and more diverse populations and to shift the emphasis from secondary and tertiary prevention towards primary prevention (Chapter 4). This represents nothing short of a major cultural transformation. Yet there is no consensus on how this might best be done or on the appropriate roles for the health professionals within PCG/Ts. Other difficult choices involve trying to improve health (which is determined by many external factors) versus improving equity of access to health services; the latter, moreover, without also incurring disproportionate efficiency costs.

The abolition of health authorities and the devolution of public health responsibilities to PCTs 3 years after the initial creation of PCGs will undoubtedly assist in the execution of this responsibility if, as suggested in Chapter 10, extensive public health expertise becomes available to, and within, PCTs. However, the lack of consensus on appropriate targets (and hence the lack of clear outcome measures and performance indicators), coupled with the long-term nature of the improvements in population health status that have been shown (Chapter 4) to be the result of primary care-based interventions, mean that any summative assessment would be premature. This is also the conclusion of Peckham in Chapter 10, following his review of the diverse initiatives and strategies so far employed by PCG/Ts in relation to health improvement.

Inequalities in the health status and the health service experiences of different sections of the population have traditionally been measured in terms of differences in mortality rates between social classes (Illsley and Le Grand 1987). This has led to the assumption that health inequalities are best countered by reductions in poverty (Townsend 1987) and in inequalities in income and housing (Rutten 1993). This is clearly not a realistic strategy for PCG/Ts. Moreover, Baker argued in Chapter 4 that health inequalities would not necessarily be reduced if the incomes of the poorest were raised, as there is little evidence that this would have a direct impact on health. Instead Baker argued that PCG/Ts should concentrate on preventive interventions targeted at conditions with social origins that are modifiable, such as anti-smoking campaigns. Other initiatives should concentrate on reducing inequalities in the take-up of screening for diseases whose early detection increases the chances of survival, such as cytology screening, although any impact on health inequalities will take some time to become apparent. Primary care trusts now also face the challenge of tackling multiple causes of inequality, including gender, age and ethnicity, as well as socio-economic status. Whether a clarity of focus can emerge from the diverse concepts, interests, strategies and activities that currently fall under the umbrella of 'health improvement' (Chapter 10) is still far from clear.

Developing primary and community health services

Although apparently unambiguous, the objective of developing primary and community health services also encompasses several different dimensions. It includes, for example, shifting the balance between hospital and primary care services in favour of the latter (Chapter 9), and improving the quality of services provided in primary care (and maintaining that improvement) (Chapter 7). In addition, the fact that virtually all PCTs have become level 4 trusts (Chapter 6) offers unprecedented opportunities to integrate the provision of primary and community health services, thereby also improving the consistency and coverage of these services. There is as yet no research evidence on how PCTs are tackling this last challenge on which their chances of success might be assessed.

According to the evidence in Chapter 7, considerable progress has been made by PCG/Ts in building the infrastructure necessary to safeguard the quality of services, despite an initial lack of clarity about the resources and mechanisms likely to be available for these tasks. However, there are also continuing tensions inherent in the clinical governance framework between those mechanisms that enhance professional self-regulation and those that rely on inspection and external regulation of quality, with the latter likely to alienate rather than engage professional involvement. The implementation of the proposed new GP contract, which is likely to contain substantial quality-related elements, will transform professional self-regulation into a contractual requirement. This increases further the risks to professional engagement in the 'modernization' process.

Commissioning

The third core function of PCG/Ts, commissioning acute and specialist services on behalf of patients, is the key through which any changes in the balance of power and command over resources between primary and secondary sectors are likely to occur. *The New NHS* (Secretary of State for Health 1997) suggested that four features should characterize the commissioning process. First, it should involve a range of stakeholders and interests, with primary care professionals at the core. According to Chapter 9, GPs' influence in commissioning predominates over that of nurses or other primary care professionals – though whether this will continue in PCTs, in which GPs no longer have a governing majority, is not clear. Secondly, in a clear retreat from the approaches of the internal market, encouragement was given to collaboration between primary care and hospital clinicians in setting appropriate quality standards and service protocols. Paradoxically, however, collaborative commissioning may reduce the 'leverage' of PCTs over hospital providers. Thirdly, national service frameworks and the treatment guidelines set by the National Institute for Clinical Excellence (NICE) were to be incorporated into commissioning processes to introduce greater consistency between local hospital services. According to Chapter 9, both national service frameworks and NICE guidelines are being used in this way, albeit to the possible detriment of locally determined priorities. Finally, it was expected that PCG/Ts might be able, over time, to improve the quality and cost-effectiveness of services by moving resources between providers. However, as Chapter 9 argued, the very large volume of services that PCTs commission, compared with fundholding GPs or total purchasing pilot projects, is likely seriously to constrain their flexibility because of the potential risk to local provider organizations. The new collaborative framework, within which commissioning now takes place, is also likely to reduce the flexibility of PCTs as commissioning bodies.

Infrastructure, partnerships and local accountability

As PCGs have become PCTs, they have required additional resources, staff and skills and appropriate organizational structures to deliver these three core functions. Chapter 6 showed that their early years were characterized by rapid expansion in both size and workload and by considerable upheaval, as PCGs merged and became trusts. It is still not certain that these capacity problems have been resolved, despite the full statutory responsibilities of PCTs and the substantial budgets that they have now assumed. Continuing shortfalls continue to be apparent in relation to the internal information management and technology (IM&T) capacity within PCTs and in their IM&T linkages with other NHS services. In contrast to the tensions apparent in other areas of PCG/T activities, between national targets and local priorities, Chapter 8 shows how the implementation of effective, high-quality IM&T systems requires strong national leadership to overcome the fragmentation and variable quality of systems that had their separate origins in general practice and other areas of the NHS. However, the shifting targets set by successive NHS IM&T strategies suggests that, realistically, this implementation will take time.

Given the poor history of collaboration between primary care and social services, and the cultural differences between these services that were revealed in the early days of the new PCG boards, considerable progress appears to have been made in relation to PCG/Ts' external partnerships. Moreover, although the focus of central government has remained almost exclusively on the relationships between PCG/Ts and social services, PCG/Ts have in fact developed much wider local networks, including links with other local statutory services and departments and participation in multi-agency initiatives such as Health Action Zones. Some of these relationships also include the transfer of resources, as PCG/Ts contribute to non-health services intended to improve the quality of life within their localities. However, other changes, particularly those in the roles, responsibilities and conditions of employment among frontline staff, that are likely to have a particular impact on the continuity experienced by service users, are more problematic; in addition, the effectiveness of PCG/Ts' partnerships may continue to be undermined by differences in geographical boundaries. Above all, strong and effective partnerships with other agencies and services need a degree of local ownership that may be difficult to sustain in the face of strengthened national targets and 'upwards' accountabilities to central government.

The New NHS: Modern, Dependable (Secretary of State for Health 1997) promised to rebuild public confidence in a NHS that is 'accountable to patients, open to the public and shaped by their views' (p. 11). However, as Chapters 6 and 11 show, there is little agreement within PCG/Ts on either the best ways or the usefulness of opening up their activities to the public. Indeed, it is possible that the introduction of new opportunities for engagement between PCG/Ts and local publics may actually come to represent the tighter management by central government of the local accountabilities of PCTs (Chapter 11). Moreover, as Chapters 2 and 5 argue, the new, explicit involvement of primary care professionals in the management of capped (albeit very large) budgets suggests the creation of new tensions arising between the interests of local populations and those of individual patients. This represents a major threat to the principal–agent relationship that has traditionally underpinned GPs' relationships with, and accountability to, their individual patients.

Modern primary care? Modern NHS?

Primary care groups/trusts are at the heart of the government's modernization programme for the NHS. They are expected to deliver improvements in access to first-contact NHS services and in the quality and integration of primary and community health services themselves. Because of the abolition of health authorities and the devolution of up to three-quarters of the total NHS budget to local levels, PCTs are now also responsible for delivering improvements in other areas of the NHS, through their commissioning activities. Indeed, the traditional boundaries of the NHS have actually been extended, through the explicit adoption of new ambitions to improve health and reduce health inequalities; PCTs are responsible for these as well.

The central role of PCTs within this system-wide 'modernization' agenda helps to explain one of the central themes that runs through this book – the tension between control and management by central government and the upwards accountabilities that accompany this, and the devolution of powers and responsibilities to local organizations in which frontline professionals and publics are actively engaged. On the face of it, the latter appears incompatible with the imperative to implement, rapidly and successfully, national policies and priorities. The contributors to this book repeatedly point to different aspects of this contradiction and its potential long-term implications.

In the pre-internal market NHS, allegedly characterized by 'centralised command and control' (Secretary of State for Health 1997: 10), this tension might have been manifest as one between managerial authority and accountability and professional autonomy and self-regulation. Indeed, despite the early introduction of general management into the hospital sector (Griffiths 1983), GPs and the services provided in their practices continued to remain relatively free from managerial authority, with the contract to provide general medical services representing the only means of state intervention and mediation in relationships between GPs and their patients (Calnan and Gabe 1991). The creation of PCG/Ts and the role of GPs within these organizations have fundamentally transformed these relationships. Through their membership of PCG/T boards, working parties and subgroups, some GPs have been fully incorporated into the management of primary care, the search for clinically effective and cost-effective services and the prioritization of expenditure within fixed budgets. The process of clinical governance extends this new mode of professional self-regulation across all local GPs and other primary care professionals, with educational strategies and joint learning events intended to strengthen collective and individual responsibilities for the quality and cost-effectiveness of their services. As the authors of Chapter 5 assert, these changes have relocated GPs to become agents of the central (rationing) state.

However, the book also points to some potential threats to the success of this distinctively 'modernizing' strategy. First, as Chapter 2 demonstrates, the conditions under which PCTs make decisions may not be conducive to consensual decision-making or to the development of trust between GPs and managers. Secondly, as Chapters 2 and 5 argue, these new roles and responsibilities may generate conflicts of interest for GPs, which may, in turn, impact on their relationships with patients. Thirdly, the attempt to integrate supportive with regulatory approaches to clinical governance, as described in Chapter 7, may also exhibit signs of strain. Fourthly, the plethora of national priorities and targets to which PCTs have increasingly had to adhere may contrast with the initial expectations of GPs and nurses of having a greater role in decision-making about local services. It may be hard to sustain their active engagement if the rhetoric of devolving responsibility to frontline professionals turns out to be little more than responsibility for implementing centrally imposed policies and targets (plus responsibility for the consequences if these targets are not met). Moreover, the managerial responsibilities of PCTs in relation to the professional practices of their constituent clinicians will only intensify in the future, with the implementation of the proposed new GP contract, as GPs and other professionals are drawn into the management of new professional quality frameworks and incentives on behalf of themselves and their peers.

This element of the NHS 'modernization' strategy appears to draw heavily on more horizontal, networked modes of governance, while simultaneously combining these with hierarchical and market modes of organization. This conflation appears potentially unstable and vulnerable to renewed fragmentation (and potential conflict) between professional and managerial interests. In the longer term, the organizational responsibilities and accountabilities of PCTs, the new GP contract and the continuing popularity of personal medical services contracts (see Chapter 1) are together likely to contribute to a fully managed primary care service. However, there may be substantial costs, both to professional morale and in relation to clinicians' relationships with their patients.

What of the other challenge that has been set PCTs, that of delivering the 'modernization' of the NHS as a whole? The substantial continuities with the former internal market – especially the continuing separation of purchasing from the provision of hospital services – provide a useful, but not very optimistic, evidence base. Moreover, some of the conditions that contributed to those aspects of the internal market that were deemed successful, particularly the capacity of GP fundholders to negotiate marginal changes in access and quality of secondary services, no longer pertain. The evidence presented in Chapter 9 suggests that collaborative relationships with secondary providers, coupled with the sheer volume of the services commissioned by PCTs, are also unlikely to offer the same opportunities for leverage as GP fundholding and total purchasing did. Moreover, there are risks that the new emphasis on preventing illness and improving health may be marginalized by shorter-term and more easily specified performance measures.

However, the evidence presented in this book, and the verdicts drawn from that evidence, need to be seen in the context of half a decade of unprecedented organizational and professional change and upheaval. Arguably, some of the most immediate consequences have been on the relationships within PCTs, between PCTs and their constituent primary and community health services and between PCTs and other local organizations. These relationships are the building blocks on which the long-term capacity and success of PCTs depend. The 'modernizing' transformation of primary care will be increasingly at risk if top-down, centrally driven agendas, directives and accountabilities lead to the alienation of frontline professionals.

For the time being, the PCT experiment remains a source of intense interest to other health care systems, which may be considerably more cautious in introducing experiments into their health services (Chapter 3). Indeed, it is arguably the eclectic 'mix' of hierarchies, markets and networks that makes the 'modernization' of the NHS so different. The risk is that overambition and impatience could render this pragmatic, but uniquely 'Third Way' combination seriously unstable.

References

Calnan, M. and Gabe, J. (1991) Recent developments in general practice: a sociological analysis, in J. Gabe, M. Calnan and M. Bury (eds) *The Sociology of the Health Service*. London: Routledge.

Crosland, A. (1956) *The Future of Socialism*. London: Cape.

Department of Health (2001) *Shifting the Balance of Power in the NHS: Securing Delivery*. London: Department of Health.

Glendinning, C., Powell, M. and Rummery, K. (2002) Partnerships, performance and primary care: developing integrated services for older people in England, *Ageing and Society*, 22(2): 185–208.

Griffiths, R. (1983) *NHS Management Inquiry Report*. London: DHSS.

Illsley, R. and Le Grand, J. (1987) The measurement of inequality in health, in A. Williams (ed.) *Health and Economics*. London: Macmillan.

Newman, J. (2001) *Modernizing Governance: New Labour, Policy and Society*. London: Sage.

Rose, N. (1996) The death of the social? Re-figuring the territory of government, *Economy and Society*, 25(3): 327–56.

Rutten, F. (1993) Policy implications of the COMAC-HSR project, in E. Van Doorslaer, A. Wagstaff and F. Rutten (eds) *Equity in the Finance and Delivery of Health Care: An International Perspective*. Oxford: Oxford University Press.

Secretary of State for Health (1997) *The New NHS: Modern, Dependable*. London: The Stationery Office.

Secretary of State for Health (2000) *The NHS Plan: A Plan for Investment, A Plan for Reform*. London: The Stationery Office.

Thompson, G., Frances, J., Levacic, R. and Mitchell, J. (eds) (1991) *Markets, Hierarchies and Networks: The Coordination of Social Life*. London: Sage.

Townsend, P. (1987) The geography of poverty and ill-health, in A. Williams (ed.) *Health and Economics*. London: Macmillan.

Index

access, 57–8
accountability, 50, 78, 80–1, 179, 180–1, 226–7
Acheson Report, 65, 160
audit, 108, 118, 127
avoidable disease/death, 60–1

Building the Information Core, 128, 129, 130

care pathways, 151
central control, 93–5
clinical governance, 101–4
causes for concern, 113–19
  causes for optimism, 112–13
  priorities, 104–5
  prospects for success, 111–19
  strategies for implementation, 105–9
clinical guidelines, 107–8
Collection of Health Data in General Practice (CHDGP), 125
collective decision-making, 29–33, 91
Commission for Health Care Audit and Inspection, 8
Commission for Health Improvement, 8, 103
Commission for Health Improvement and Assessment, 103
Commission for Patient and Public Involvement in Health, 184–5
commissioning, 225–7
  influences on priorities, 147–9
  partnerships, 203–4
  performance of PCGs/PCTs, 149–52
    variations, 152–4
  responsibility for, 146–7
  shifting the balance, 142, 145
  v. purchasing, 144–6
  vertical integration, 74–5
communities, 172–3
community governance, 27–36
community health councils, 181
complexity, 91–3
consultative bodies, 31
contradiction, 228
cooperation, 25–7

coronary heart disease, 113–14
corporacy, 29, 36, 112
culture, 32, 112, 145, 163, 224

Delivering, 21st Century Support for the NHS, 128–9, 131, 139
Delivering the NHS Plan, 25
democracy, 180–1
democratic accountability, 179–94
Denmark, 44
dictatorial decision-making, 30–2
disciplinary procedures, 109–10
distribution, 54–9
doctor involvement, 190
doctor-patient relationship, risks, 70–81

education, 106–7
efficiency/equity trade-off, 63
electronic health record, 137
electronic patient records, 137
equity/inequity, 54–66
evaluating performance, 223–5
executive councils, 180
experimentation, 51–2

family practitioner committees, 181
financial framework, 95–8
Finland, 42–3, 50, 52
Fit for the Future, 9
France, 41, 58
frontline partnerships, 205–6
fundholders/fundholding, 12–14, 23, 150, 181

game theory, 36
gender, 58, 64
general medical services contracts, 79–80
general practice, 11–15, 118, 124
Germany, 41–2
governance, 22, 27–36, 85–99, 101–19
GP contracts, 78–80, 126, 222, 225

health authorities, 10, 180–1
health care distribution, 54–9

health distribution, 58–9
health improvement, 160, 168–73, 224–5
Health in Partnership initiative, 193–4
hierarchies, 221–3
horizontal equity, 55

ideology and performance, 219–30
incentive schemes, 57, 107, 113, 151
Independent Inquiry into Inequalities in Health
    (Acheson), 65
inequalities, 54–66, 224
Information for Health, 127–31, 137
information systems, 123–39
    development in primary care, 124–7, 174
    progress and challenges, 133–8
    role of primary health organisations, 132–3
    strategic vision, 127–31
inter-agency partnerships, 206–8
internal market, 11–15, 43, 144, 231
    see also quasi-markets
inverse equity, 57, 61–2
Involving Patients and the Public in Health Care,
    182
Italy, 48

Jarman Index, 56
joint activities, 205

local accountability, 50, 226–7
local authorities, 208–9
local autonomy, 93–5
local health improvement, 168–73
local involvement, 186–7
local responsibility, 25–7

manager involvement, 190–1
managerial responsibilities, 228–9
markets, 221–2
mergers, 91–2
micro-management techniques, 50–1
modernization, 3–11, 21, 219, 227–30

National Electronic Library for Health, 135
National Health Service Act 1946, 180
The National Institute for Clinical
    Excellence, 8, 102–3
national service frameworks, 102
national targets, 32
needs assessment, 56–7
Netherlands, 49, 60
networks, 27, 221, 223
New Labour, 3–11, 21, 182–5

New NHS, 23–4
The New NHS: Modern, Dependable (White
    Paper, 1997), 5–8, 11, 21, 25–6, 70, 86,
    145–6, 219–21, 223, 226–7
New Zealand, 44–6, 52, 60
NHS models, 220
NHS net, 135, 137
*The NHS Plan: A Plan for Investment, A Plan for
    Reform*, 9–10, 128–30, 135, 139, 146,
    164, 221
Nordic countries, 42–4
Northern Ireland, 8–9
Norway, 43–4

organizational aspects, 24–9, 86–9, 98–9, 172
overview and scrutiny committees, 183–4
ownership, 22

Partnership in Action, 199
partnerships, 226–7
    definitions and rationales, 196–8
    history, 198
    inter-agency, 206–8
    local, 196–212
    new agenda, 199–200
    problems and barriers, 208–12
    public health, 170–1
patient advice and liaison services, 183
patient choice, 49–50
patient involvement, 182–3, 186–91, 223
Patient and Public Involvement in the New NHS,
    182
Patient Representation in the New NHS, 182
performance, 109–11
    evaluating, 223–5
    ideology and, 219–30
    poor, systems for dealing with, 109–11
personal medical services contracts, 14, 79
pilot schemes, 51–2
planning, 180–1, 203–4
policy innovations, 15–16
population need, 55
preventive interventions, 60–4, 225
primary care, 48–9, 219–20, 224
    and public health, 162–4
primary care groups/trusts
    institutional development, 23–4
    international experience, 48–9
    Labour's reforms (modernization), 6–11
    local health improvement, 168–73
    organizational aspects, 24–9, 87–9, 98–9,
        172

policy and guidance, 161–2
public health, 162–8
vertical integration, 75–6
Primary Care Information Modernization Programme, 130
Primary Care Information Services (PRIMIS), 126, 134
primary v. secondary care, 142–56
principal-agent models, 71–4, 77, 222, 227
Priorities and Planning Framework 2003–2006, 174
Private Finance Initiative, 22
professional ethics, 76, 80
provision, vertical integration, 74–5
public health, 59–60, 159–75
public involvement, 182–91
purchasing, 143–4
v. commissioning, 144–6

quality of health care, improvement, 101–19
quality standards, 151
quasi-markets, 145–6, 149, 154, 198

reforms, 5–11
Russian Federation, 48

Saving Lives: Our Healthier Nation, 159, 161–2
Scotland, 8–9
seamless services, 205, 211, 222
secondary v. primary care, 142–56
service integration, 50–1
service level agreements, 150
shifting the balance of power, 142–56
Shifting the Balance of Power in the NHS, 10, 87, 93–4, 138, 146, 161, 222

social services, 198–9, 205, 227
social services representative, 200–3, 206–8, 210
Spain, 48, 58
special project approaches, 171–2
stakeholders, 89–91, 182–91, 223
standards, 107–8, 151
strategic health authorities, 87
success, criteria for, 15–18
Sweden, 43–4

targets
central government, 32
health improvement, 168
information agenda, 128–9, 131, 135–8
service commissioning, 151
telemedicine, 135, 137
Third Way
New Labour philosophy, 4–5, 21–2, 220–1
weaknesses, 27, 37, 230
total purchasing, 25, 74, 198
Tracker Survey, 17–18
training, 106–7
trust, 33–6
two-tier system, 150

unified budgets, 26–7, 77, 93, 95
USA, 21, 46–9, 52

vertical equity, 55
vertical integration, 74–6

Wales, 8–9
Wanless Report, 130
welfare advice, 171

REASONABLE RATIONING
INTERNATIONAL EXPERIENCE OF PRIORITY SETTING IN HEALTH CARE

Chris Ham and Glenn Robert (Eds.)

Reasonable Rationing is must reading for those interested in how to connect theory about fair rationing processes to country-level practices. The five case studies reveal a deep tension between political pressures to accommodate interest group demands and ethically motivated efforts to improve both information and institutional procedures for setting fair limits to care. The authors frame the issues insightfully.

Professor Norman Daniels, Harvard School of Public Health

- How are different countries setting priorities for health care?
- What role does information and evidence on cost and effectiveness play?
- How are institutions contributing to priority setting?
- What are the lessons for policy makers?

Priority setting in health care is an issue of increasing importance. Choices about the use of health care budgets are inescapable and difficult. A number of countries have sought to strengthen their approach to priority setting by drawing on research-based evidence on the cost and effectiveness of different treatments. This book brings together leading experts in the field to summarize and analyse the experience of priority setting in five countries: Canada, The Netherlands, New Zealand, Norway and the United Kingdom. Drawing on literature from a range of disciplines, it makes a significant contribution to the debate on the role of information and institutions in priority setting.

Reasonable Rationing has been written with a broad readership in mind. It will be of interest to policy makers, health care professionals and health service managers, as well as students of health and social policy at advanced undergraduate and postgraduate levels.

Contents
Introduction – International experience of rationing – New Zealand – Canada – United Kingdom – Norway – The Netherlands – Conclusions – References – Index.

192pp   0 335 21185 2 (Paperback)   0 335 21186 0 (Hardback)

CONTEMPORARY PRIMARY CARE
THE CHALLENGES OF CHANGE
Philip Tovey (ed)

Primary care is currently going through a period of substantial change. The high profile alteration of structures is occurring at a time when many issues of practice are presenting new or renewed challenges. These are issues grounded in the complexities and dissatisfactions of contemporary society as well as in the changing policy context.

This book has been produced in order to bring together critical and thought-provoking pieces on these wide-ranging challenges, by authors from an equally wide range of disciplines, including anthropology, clinical psychology, disability studies, public health, sociology, as well as general practice.

Beginning with a think piece on the nature of primary care and what an emerging vision for it might look like, the book continues with contributions on the changing form, organization and delivery of primary health care, before going on to examine specific areas of provision and some significant research issues. The book will be of interest to all those involved in the study or development of primary health care services.

Contents
Introduction – Part one: Challenges of context and organization – Vision and change in primary care: past, present and future – The changing character of service provision – The changing nature of primary health care teams and inter-professional relationships – Part two: Challenges of practice – Commissioning services for older people: make haste slowly? – Disability: from medical needs to social rights – The new genetics and general practice: revolution or continuity? – Socio-economic inequality: beyond the inverse care law – Part three: Challenges of research – Locality planning and research evidence: using primary care data – Counselling: researching an evidence base for practice – Complementary medicine and primary care: towards a grassroots focus – Postscript – Index

192pp   0 335 20009 5 (Paperback)   0 335 20452 X (Hardback)